Eating Light
SOUS VIDE COOKBOOK

Discover the Best Light, Tasty, and Budget-Friendly Sous Vide Recipes to Prepare Perfect Meals for Your Whole Family. Perfect for Everyone from Beginner to Advanced.

Sophia Marchesi

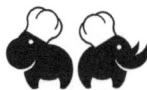

IPPOCERONTE
publishing

Cover designed by thiwwy design (@thiwwy).
Cover Photo by Ella Olsson (@ellaolsson) from Unsplash

CONTENTS

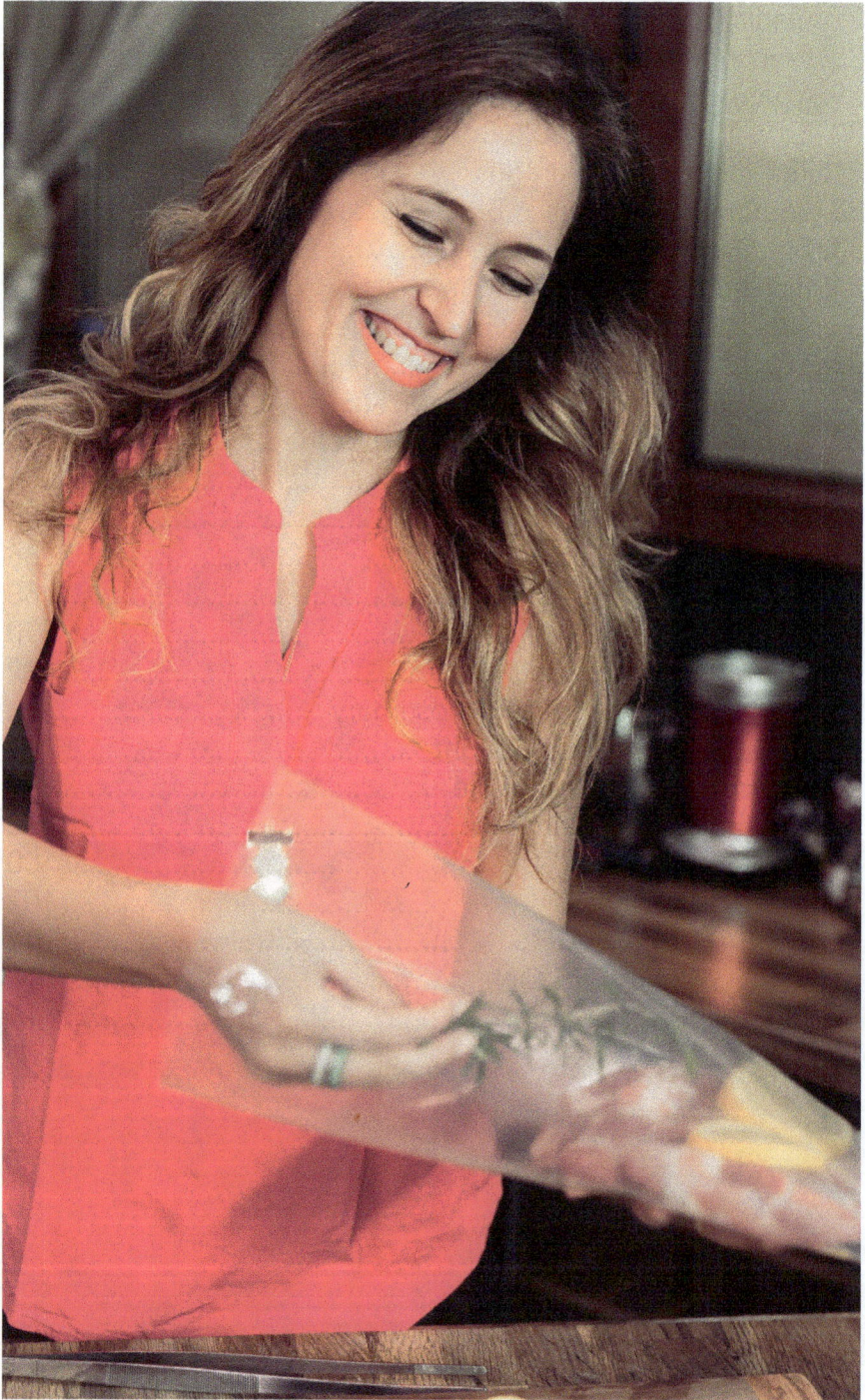

INTRODUCTION

In this book, I have collected a selection of my favorite light recipes, some are re-elaborations of classic recipes that I used to do with my family when I was younger, others are the result of my travels around the world. Each recipe in this book evokes a memory of an important moment in my life, so I hope you will enjoy them.

Cooking is something that runs in my blood, most of my food memories are of my Nan cooking Sunday dinners - lasagna and cannelloni to share with the whole family. When I was young, I have never liked to be stuck in a classroom, I started culinary school at a very young age, and the only thing I really wanted was to be out cooking. You could say I was not a particularly good student, but I have always been really passionate about food.

I have been working in a professional kitchen since I was seventeen years old and I'm running my own restaurant since I was 23. The past thirty years have been a rewarding, yet arduous journey that I spent learning the basics and mastering the different cuisines and techniques by taking the best out of each of them. It was last year, during the lockdown, that I realized that I was starting to lose my passion. Preparing a dish had become an aseptic and mechanical where perfection was king.

I wanted to go back to my roots, cooking has always been about my family; preparing a dish together with the people I love gives me time to connect and create precious memories. Setting aside a time where the entire family can work together to create a meal gives us a chance to pause, catch up and just connect with each other.

What I would like to share with you in this book is my renewed passion and a technique that I learned during my time in France, the Sous Vide. This innovative cooking method is something my grandmother never thought existed and creates the perfect opportunity to spend some time in the kitchen with my family. For these reasons, I think the Sous Vide is the perfect combination of my professional and domestic life.

Sous Vide is the French term that translates to "under vacuum" and it is the method for preparing a dish at a specifically controlled temperature and time; your food should be prepared at the temperature at which it will be eaten. Put simply, this procedure involves placing food in vacuum seal bags and boiling it in a specially built bath of water for longer than average cooking times (usually 1 to 7 hours, up to 48 or more in some cases). Cooking at an exact temperature takes the guesswork out of the equation that defines a perfect meal. You can easily prepare your steak, chicken, lamb, pork, etc., exactly the way you like it, every single time.

It is easy to use and leads to great results every time. You will end up with food that is more tender and juicier than anything else you've ever made. This technique will help you to take your everyday cooking to a higher level. To do a top dish, most of the time, you do not need exotic ingredients, it is just a matter to get the best from the ingredients you already know.

The greatest part of Sous Vide cooking is that it does not require your constant presence in the kitchen. When the food is sealed in a bag and placed in the water bath, you can leave it at a low temperature, and it will cook on its own without asking much of your attention. The Sous Vide Cookers that are nowadays available in the market are efficient at regulating the perfect temperature to cook food according to its texture while maintaining the minimum required temperature. So, while your food is in the water, your hands are practically free to work on other important tasks or spend some quality time with your family.

It is an artful skill that is definitely worth trying. If it is just your first time, don't feel bad if you don't get the results you wanted to achieve. You will get better by gaining experience with this cookbook! The key is having patience, the right information, and consistency.

The meals prepared with Sous Vide are tasty and healthy, since this technique does not use added fats during the preparation of your dish also, using low temperature ensures that the perfect cooking point is reached.

Dishes included in this cookbook are simple, delicious, and provide you with so many options that you'll be preparing them for years to come. These recipes are made to be shared with the people you love and to build new precious food memories as I did with my Nan.

RECIPES

1. OVERNIGHT OATMEAL

Cal.: 284 | Fat: 20g | Protein: 9g

Preparation Time: 11 minutes
Cooking Time: 10 hours
Servings: 4

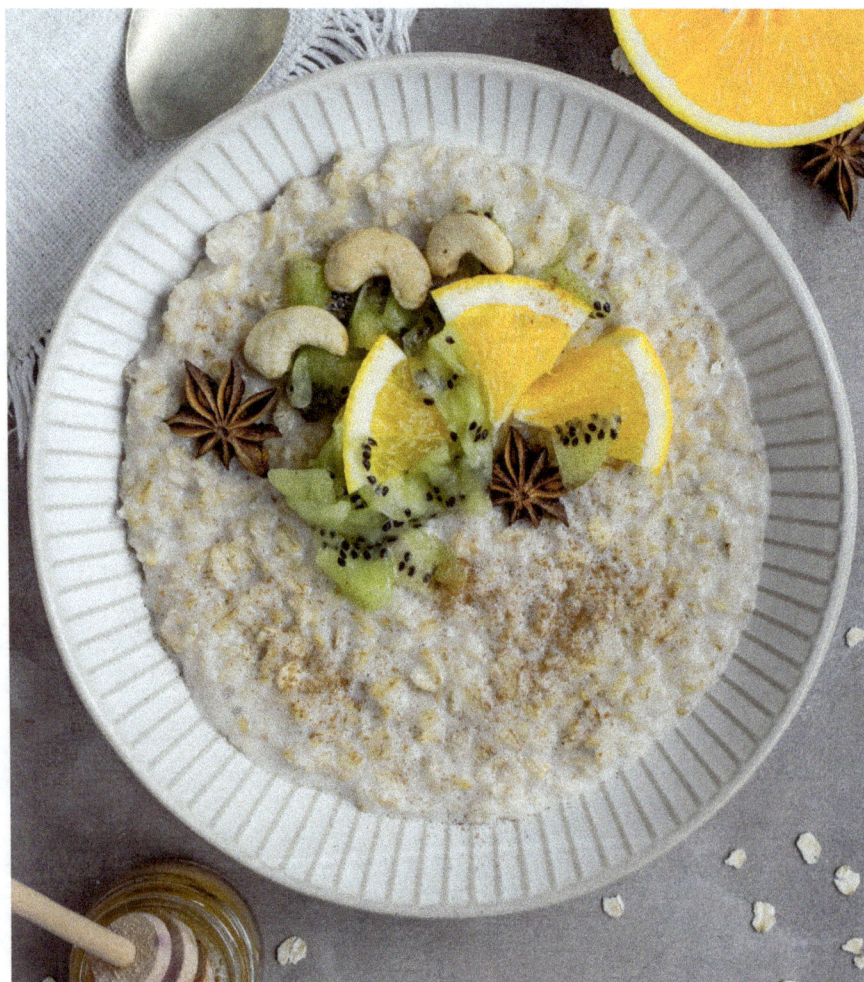

Ingredients

2/3 cup rolled oats
2/3 cup pinhead oatmeal
1 1/3 cups milk or cream
4 teaspoons raisins
2 cups water
2 teaspoons maple syrup or honey

Directions

1. Preheat the Sous Vide machine to 140°F/60°C.

2. Take 4 Mason jars or glass jam jars with lids. Divide the oats and pinhead oatmeal (you can also use quick-cook steel-cut oats) among the jars. Divide the milk and pour over the oats. Pour ½ cup water in each jar.

3. Add a teaspoon of raisins to each jar. Fasten the lids lightly, not tight.

4. Immerse the filled jars in the water bath. The lids of the jars should be above the level of water in the cooker. This is important.

5. Set the timer for 9 to 10 hours.

6. When done, stir and serve with some butter, if desired.

2. CHICKEN NOODLE SOUP

Cal.: 366 | Fat: 29g | Protein: 15g

Preparation Time: 13 minutes
Cooking Time: 60 minutes
Servings: 2

Ingredients

3 pounds whole chicken, trussed
3 cups carrots, finely diced
9 cups chicken stock
3 cups white onion, finely diced
3 cups celery, finely diced
Salt to taste
Pepper to taste
2 bay leaves
1 ½ pounds dried egg noodles

Directions

1. Set your Sous Vide machine to 150°F/65°C.

2. Add all the ingredients, except noodles, into a large Ziploc bag or a vacuum-seal bag. Remove all the air with the water displacement method or a vacuum-sealed. Seal and Immerse the bag in the water bath and cook for 6 hours or until the vegetables and chicken are cooked. Cover the

cooker with plastic wrap so that the evaporation is kept to the minimum.

3. When done, remove from the cooker. Transfer into a large pot. Place the pot over medium heat.

4. Cook for around 20 minutes. Remove the chicken with a slotted spoon.

5. Add noodles and cook until al dente. Shred the chicken with a pair of forks and add it back into the pot.

6. Heat thoroughly and serve.

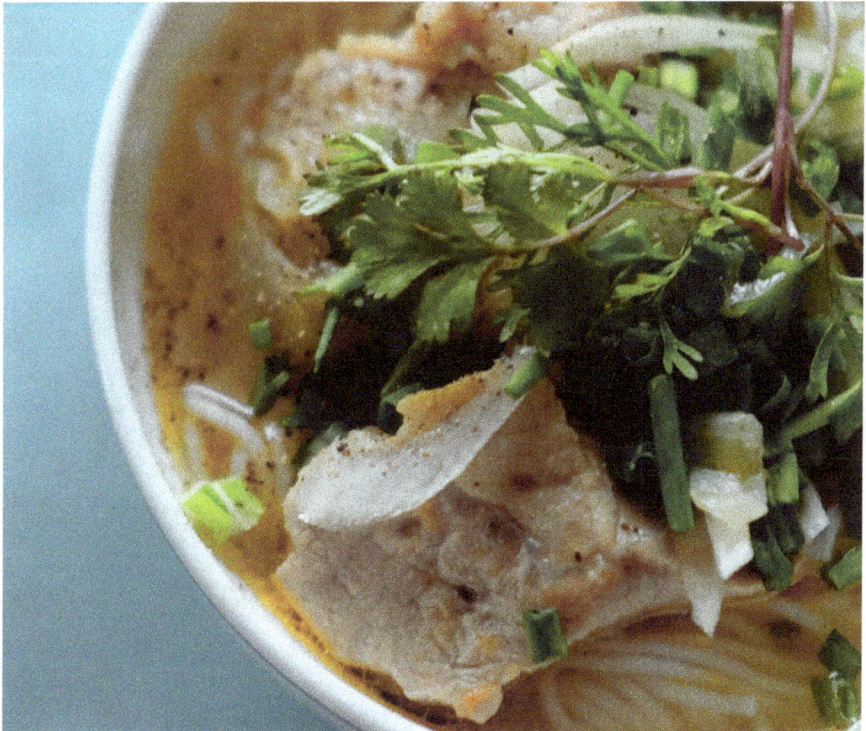

3. CHILI SHRIMP SOUP

Cal.: 127 | Fat: 8g | Protein: 23g

Preparation Time: 10 minutes
Cooking Time: 60 minutes
Servings: 1

Ingredients

1 lb. shrimps
1 onion
2 carrots
1 bell pepper
1 yellow zucchini
3 garlic cloves
3 celery stalks
2 teaspoon chili powder
1 tablespoon olive oil
1 cup chicken broth
1 cup tomato juice
½ cup corn kernels
Salt, pepper, oregano as per taste

Directions

1. Heat oil in a pan and cook all the vegetables for 3 minutes.

2. Add all the spices, broth and tomatoes. Simmer for

20 minutes.

3. Preheat the Sous Vide machine to 195°F/91°C.

4. Take the shrimps in a Ziploc bag and apply a vacuum to remove the air.

5. Place this bag in the water bath for 30 minutes.

6. The shrimps should turn pink.

7. Add the shrimps to the above pan and cook for 2 minutes.

8. Garnish with the lime wheels and serve hot.

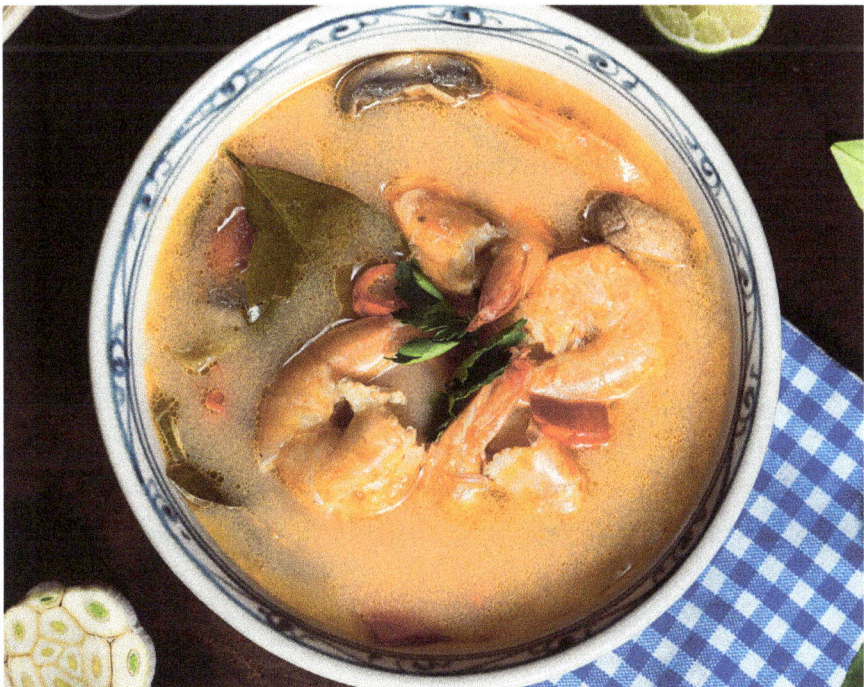

4. CHEESY BROCCOLI SOUP

Cal.: 200 | Fat: 3g | Protein: 4g

Preparation Time: 15 minutes
Cooking Time: 30 minutes
Servings: 4

Ingredients

5 tablespoons butter
1 chopped onion
1 cup chopped celery
3 minced garlic cloves
¼ cup flour
8 cup vegetable broth
5 cup broccoli florets
1 chopped carrot
3 cups shredded cheddar cheese
Salt and pepper

Directions

1. In a cooking bowl, melt butter and cook the onion and garlic.

2. Add broth, salt, pepper and boil until thicken.

3. Preheat the Sous Vide machine to 175°F/79°C.

4. Take the broccoli florets and chopped cabbage in the Ziploc bag and vacuum seal it.

5. Place the bag in and cook for 20 minutes.

6. Add the cooked broccoli and cook for 2 minutes.

7. Make a purée of this mixture.

8. Take this purée in a bowl, add cheese and heat for 1 minute.

9. Serve hot.

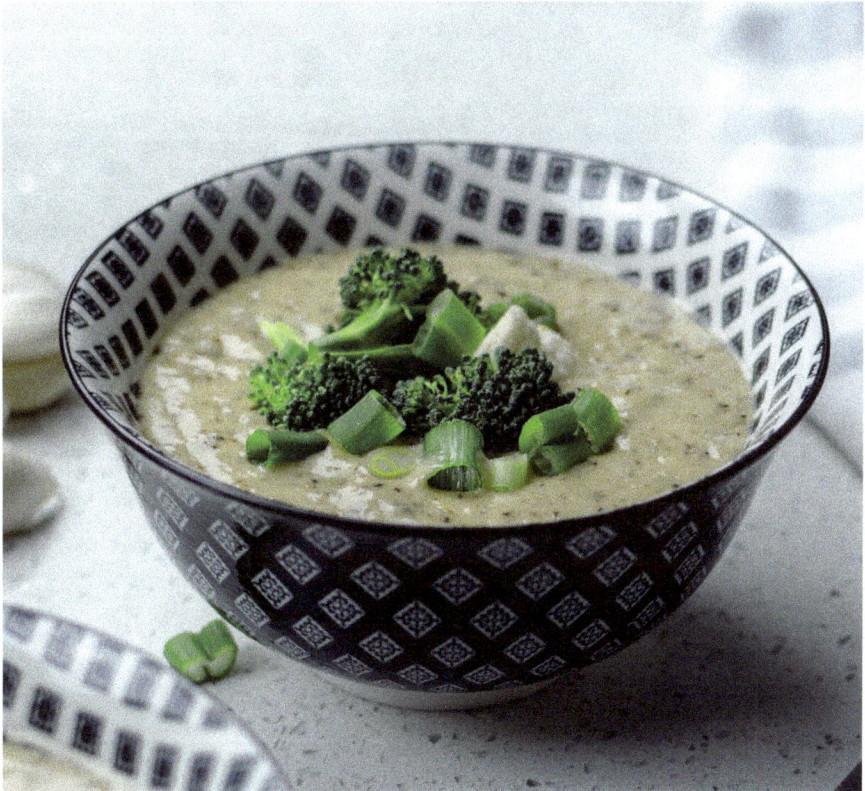

5. MUSHROOM SOUP

Cal.: 254 | Fat: 21.7g | Protein: 3.6g

Preparation Time: 50 minutes
Cooking Time: 2 hours 40 minutes
Servings: 3

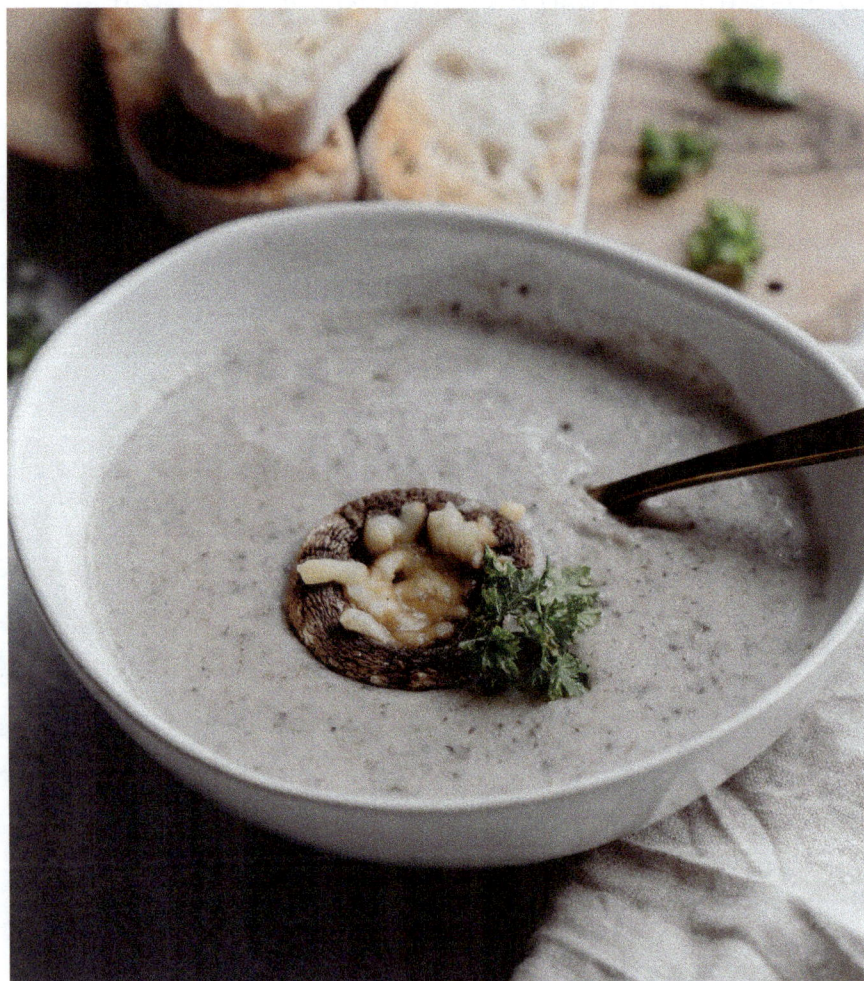

Ingredients

1 lb. mixed mushrooms
2 onions, diced
3 garlic cloves
2 sprigs parsley leaves, chopped
2 tbsp. thyme powder
2 tbsp. olive oil
2 cups cream
2 cups vegetable stock

Directions

1. Make a water bath, place it, and set to 185°F/85°C. Place the mushrooms, onion, and celery in a vacuum-sealable bag. Release air by the water displacement method, seal and Immerse the bag in the water bath. Set the timer for 30 minutes. Once the timer has stopped, remove and unseal the bag.

2. Blend the ingredients in the bag in a blender. Put a pan over medium heat, add the olive oil. Once it starts to heat, add the pureed mushrooms and the remaining listed ingredients, except for the cream. Cook for 10 minutes. Turn off heat and add cream. Stir well. Serve.

6. SALMON MARINATED IN MAPLE SYRUP

Cal.: 469 | Fat: 34g | Protein: 18g

Preparation Time: 8 minutes
Cooking Time: 51 minutes
Servings: 4

Ingredients

One salmon loin of approximately 150 g, around 2.5 cm thick
Salt, to taste
Pepper, to taste
1 sprig of dill
25g maple syrup
1 potato
1 small aubergine (eggplant)
½ a red pepper
50 ml white wine
Extra virgin olive oil to taste

Directions

1. Preheat the water bath to 149°F/65°C.

2. Salt and pepper the salmon to taste and put it into a vacuum bag together with the dill and maple syrup.

---

3. Seal the bag and place in a water bath.

4. Cut the aubergine, potato and pepper into small cubes and toss it with a drop of oil and the white wine.

5. When the salmon is finished, take it out and open the bag.

6. Reserve the cooking liquids.

7. To serve: place the vegetables on the plate and the salmon on top, dress it and finish it off with a dash of extra virgin olive oil.

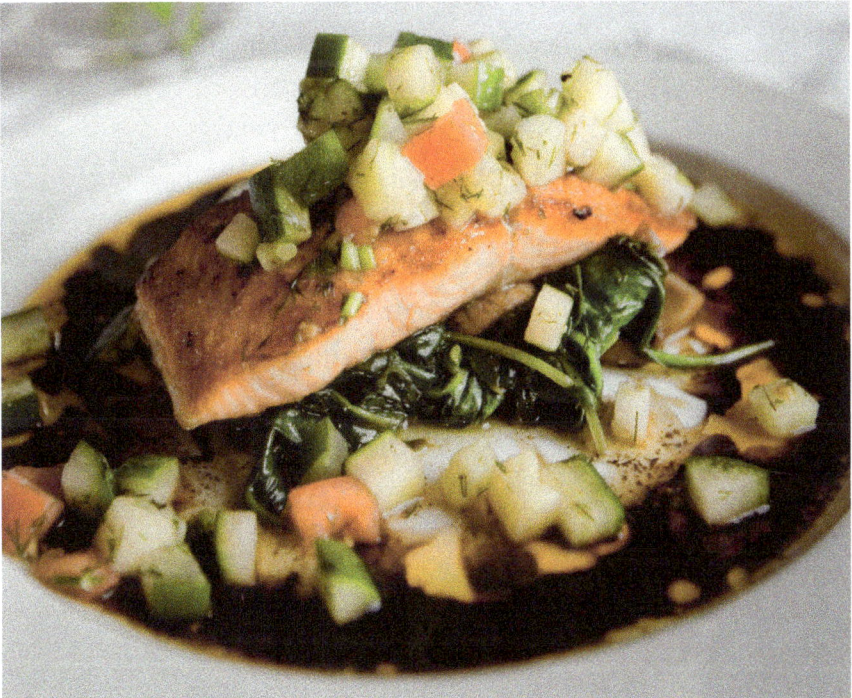

7. PICKLED SHRIMPS

Cal.: 120 | Fat: 4.5g | Protein: 13g

Preparation Time: 15 minutes
Cooking Time: 30 minutes
Servings: 8

Ingredients

1 tablespoon fennel seeds
1 teaspoon coriander seeds
1 teaspoon thyme
1 teaspoon cilantro
½ teaspoon oregano
½ tablespoon mustard seeds
2 tablespoon olive oil
1 teaspoon lemon zest
1-pound shrimps
2 oz. garlic cloves, peeled
1 tablespoon bay leaf
3 tablespoon vinegar
¼ cup lime juice
1 white onion
1 teaspoon salt

Directions

1. Peel the onion and grate it. Combine the grated onion, lemon zest, lime juice and vinegar in a large bowl. Add peeled shrimps. Season with fennel seeds, coriander seeds, thyme, cilantro, oregano, mustard seeds, salt and olive oil. Stir to combine well.

2. Transfer the mixture to a plastic bag and seal it.

3. Preheat the Sous Vide machine to 149°F/65°C and cook the shrimps for 30 minutes.

4. When ready, Serve and enjoy!

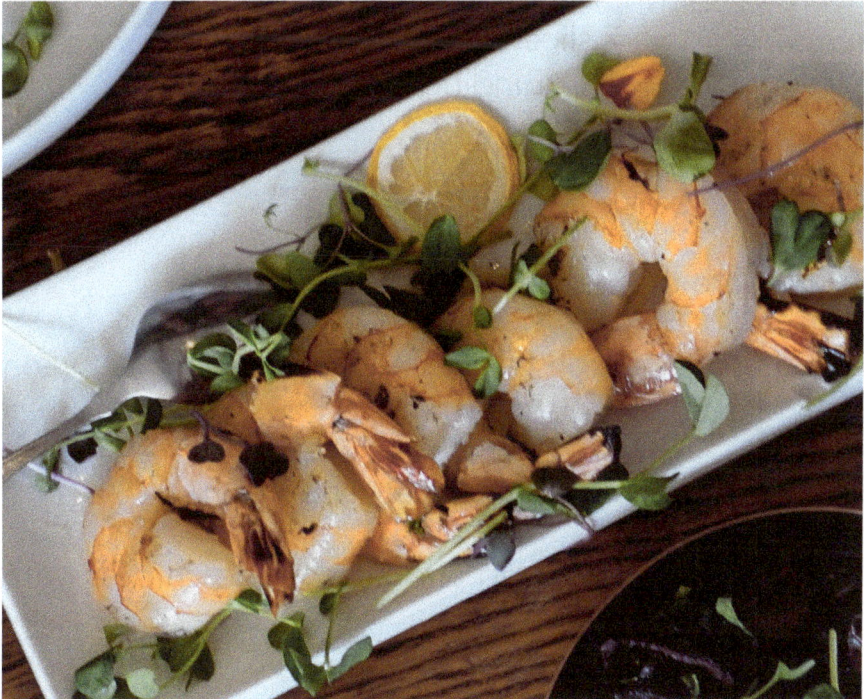

8. EASY CHICKEN CORDON BLEU

Cal.: 276 | Fat: 14g | Protein: 34.2g

Preparation Time: 6 minutes
Cooking Time: 90 minutes
Servings: 4

Ingredients

2 boneless, skinless chicken breasts
1 teaspoon sea salt
1 teaspoon black pepper
4 Swiss cheese slices
2 slices of uncured ham
Binding string

Directions

1. Prepare the water bath to 140°F/60°C.

2. Butterfly chicken breasts and place them between two sheets of plastic wrap.

3. Tenderize flat using a meat tenderizer.

4. Remove plastic wrap and season the chicken with salt and pepper.

5. Lay Swiss cheese in a single layer down the middle of each chicken breast.

6. Place a layer of uncured ham on top of the cheese.

7. Roll each chicken breast up like a jelly roll, beginning at the narrowest edge. Use a binding string on each end to hold together.

8. Place the chicken rolls in a vacuum bag, seal and cook for 1 hour 30 minutes.

9. Allow chicken to rest for 5 minutes, and slice to serve warm.

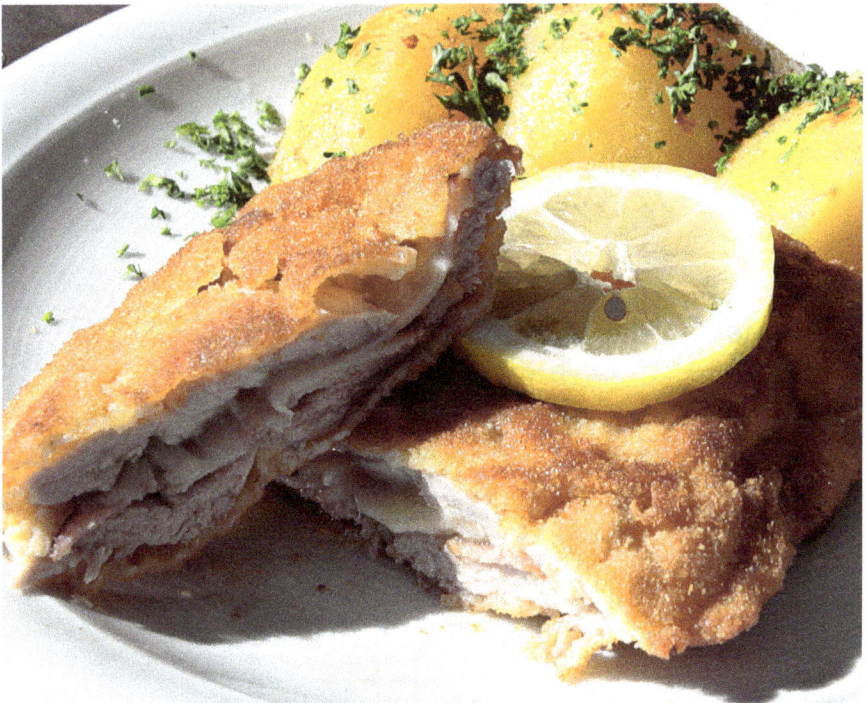

9. SALMON BURGER

Cal.: 138 | Fat: 6g | Protein: 18g

Preparation Time: 10 minutes
Cooking Time: 30 minutes
Servings: 4

Ingredients

2 cups salmon
2 ½ cup bread crumbs
3 eggs
3/4 cup celery
1 cup green onions
2 tablespoons oil
4 English muffins
Salt, pepper, fries as per need

Directions

1. Preheat the Sous Vide machine to 195°F/91°C.

2. Take the salmon in a bag and apply a vacuum to remove the air.

3. Place this bag in the water bath for 10 minutes.

4. Take a large bowl and beat the eggs.

5. Add the cooked salmon, bread crumbs, celery, green onions, salt, pepper and mix.

6. Make 4 patties from the above dough and cook in oil for 10 minutes on medium flame. Flip and repeat.

7. Place the patty on the toasted English muffin and garnish with favorite salads.

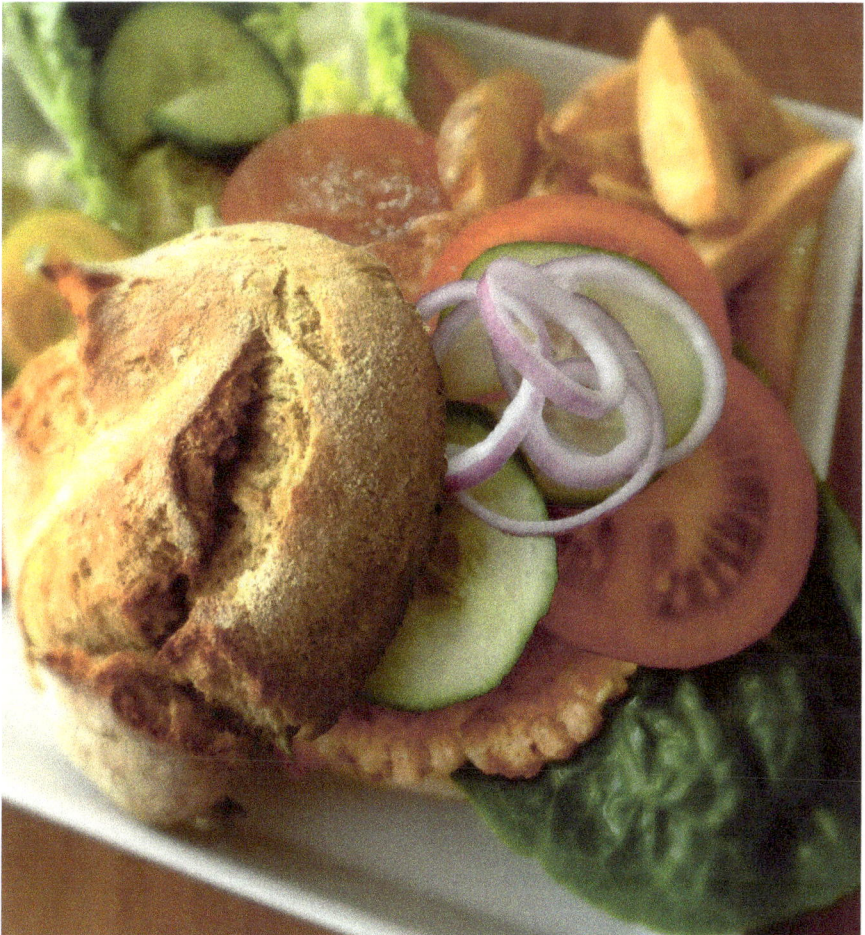

10. CLAMS WITH WHITE WINE AND ARTICHOKE HEARTS

Cal.: 158 | Fat: 10.3g | Protein: 8.6g

Preparation Time: 31 minutes
Cooking Time: 11 minutes
Servings: 4

Ingredients

24 clams
1 cup marinated artichoke hearts
3 garlic cloves
2 tbsp. extra virgin olive oil
1 tablespoon cornstarch
1 cup veggie or fish stock
3 tbsp. white wine
Salt and pepper to taste
Parsley for garnish

Directions

1. Preheat the Sous Vide machine to 133°F/56°C. Rinse the clams, slice the garlic, and cut the hearts in half.

2. Place the stock and wine in a pot and heat it on high heat until it boils. Place the clams in the boiling pot until they open.

3. Remove the clams from the pot and allow to cool for 15 minutes.

4. Place the cooled ingredients in a bag with the garlic and olive oil and place the bag in your preheated container for 3 minutes. While the clams are cooking, heat a skillet over medium heat.

5. When the clams are cooked, transfer the liquid to the heated skillet. Mix in the cornstarch until the sauce thickens. Add in the artichoke heart until they're warm. Then mix in the clams for a few seconds before removing from heat. Serve in bowls topped with parsley.

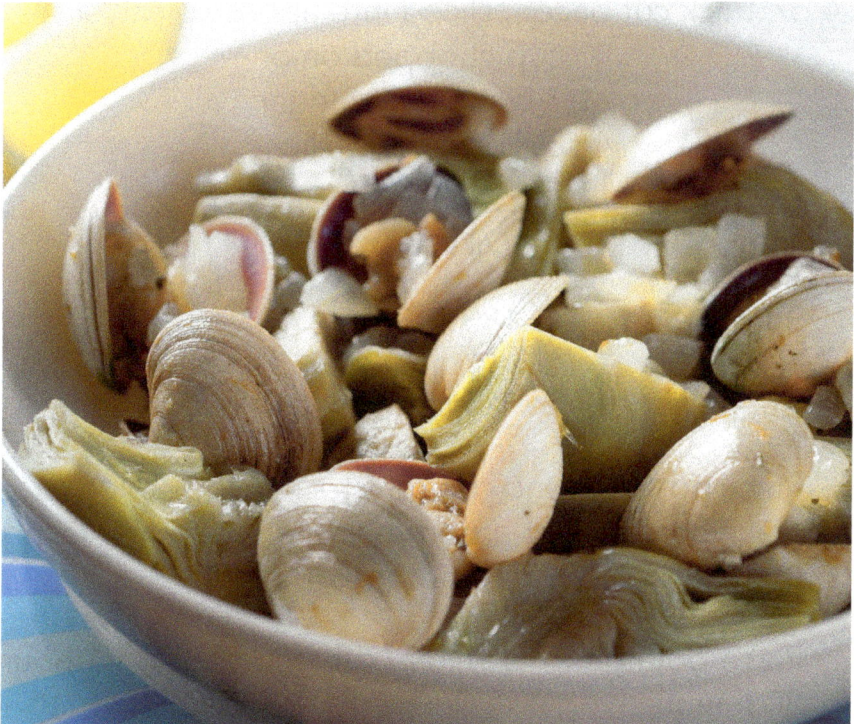

11. POTATO SALAD

Cal.: 108 | Fat: 1.6g | Protein: 3.7g

Preparation Time: 11 minutes
Cooking Time: 90 minutes
Servings: 6

Ingredients

1 ½ pounds yellow potatoes or red potatoes (waxy
potatoes work best)
½ cup chicken stock
Salt and pepper to taste
4 oz. thick cut bacon, sliced into about ¼-inch slices
½ cup chopped onion
1/3 cup cider vinegar
4 scallions, thinly sliced

Directions

1. Set the cooker to 185°F/85°C.

2. Cut potatoes into ¾-inch-thick cubes.

3. Place potatoes and chicken stock to the Ziploc bag,
   making sure they are in a single layer; seal using
   the immersion water method.

4. Place potatoes in a water bath and cook for 1 hour
   30 minutes.

5. Meanwhile, in the last 15 minutes, heat the non-stick skillet over medium-high heat. Add bacon and cook until crisp; remove bacon and add chopped onions. Cook until softened for 5-7 minutes.

6. Add vinegar and cook until reduced slightly.

7. Remove potatoes from the water bath and place them in a skillet, with the cooking water.

8. Continue cooking for a few minutes until the liquid thickens.

9. Remove potatoes from the heat and stir in scallions; toss to combine.

10.   Serve while still hot.

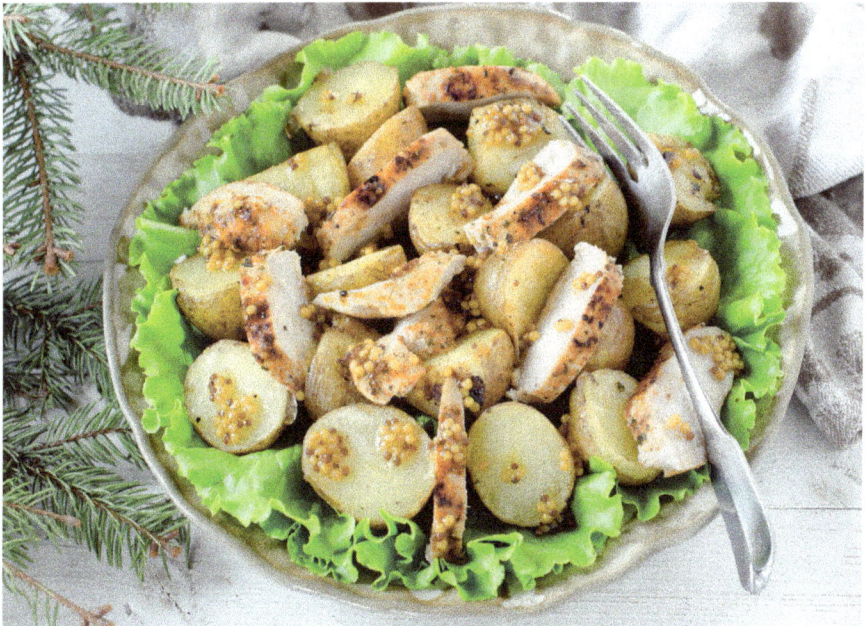

12. SAFFRON CLEMENTINE

Cal.: 300 | Fat: 12.5g | Protein: 4g

Preparation Time: 20 minutes
Cooking Time: 6 hours
Servings: 8

Ingredients

4 whole clementines, peeled
3/4 cup honey
1/4 teaspoon allspice, ground
2 crushed cardamom seeds
1 pinch saffron
Zest of 2 clementines
2 bay leaves
½ cinnamon stick
1 cup brown sugar
2 cups double cream
2 ½ cups milk
1/4 teaspoon ground nutmeg
½ cup sugar

Directions

1. Prepare and preheat the water bath at 185°F/85°C.

2. Add clementines and all the ingredients to a zipper-lock bag.

3. Seal the zipper-lock bag using the water immersion method.

4. Place the sealed bag in the bath and cook for 6 hours.

5. Once done, transfer the clementines to a plate and cut them in half.

6. Strain the remaining liquid and pour it over the clementines.

7. Serve.

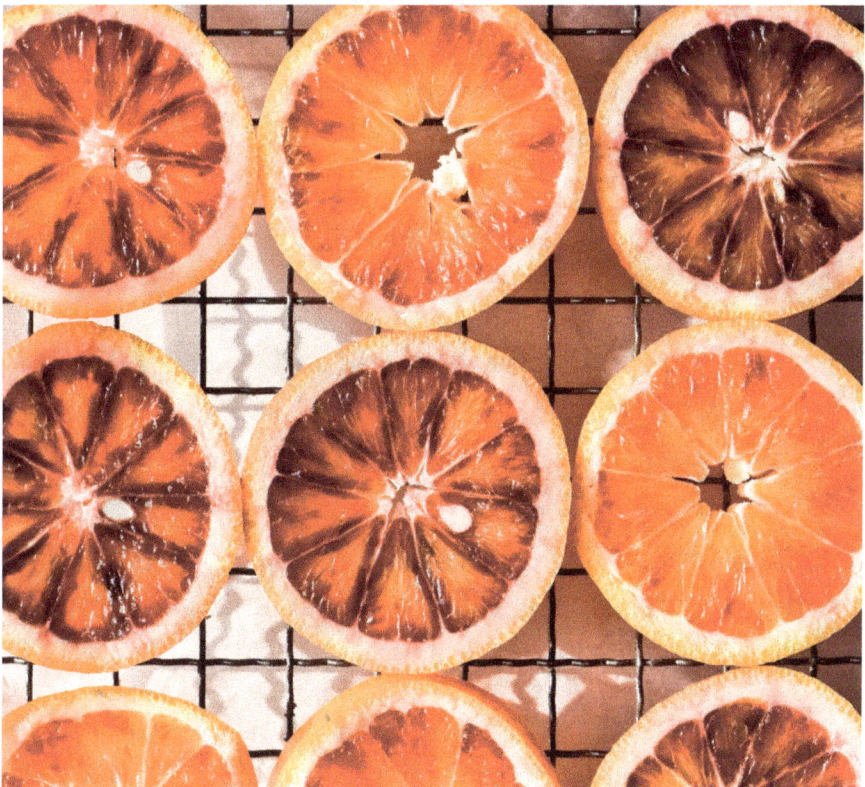

13. TOMATOES WITH SHEEP CHEESE

Cal.: 369 | Fat: 23g | Protein: 14g

Preparation Time: 9 minutes
Cooking Time: 31 minutes
Servings: 2

Ingredients

400 g sheep cheese
700 g beef tomatoes
350 g colorful cocktail tomatoes
1 tbsp. olive oil
1 handful of basil leaves
2 sprigs of thyme and 2 sprigs of rosemary each
1 chili pepper
2 garlic cloves
1 tsp. sugar
Pepper and sea salt

Directions

1. Place cocktail tomatoes in boiling water for 1 minute, then pour off the water and peel off the skin of the tomatoes.

2. Roast a finely-diced garlic with the same chili in a pan in 1 tablespoon of olive oil.

3. Finely purée the beefsteak tomatoes with garlic, chili and a little sea salt. Obtain the clear tomato stock by pressing the tomato mixture through a paper towel.

4. Put in a suitable vacuum bag: the cherry tomatoes with the tomato stock, the remaining clove of garlic, the herbs, sugar and olive oil.

5. Vacuum seal.

6. Preheat the water bath to 176°F/80°C and cook the tomato bag for 20 minutes.

7. In the meantime, bake the sheep's cheese in an oven preheated to 356°F/180°C until it is soft. This takes about 15 minutes. Then it has a light tan.

8. Open the bag carefully. Spread the sheep's cheese on two plates. Add the cocktail tomatoes with their sauce.

14. GREEN BEAN ALMONDINE

Cal.: 294 | Fat: 20g | Protein: 13g

Preparation Time: 8 minutes
Cooking Time: 1 hour
Servings: 4

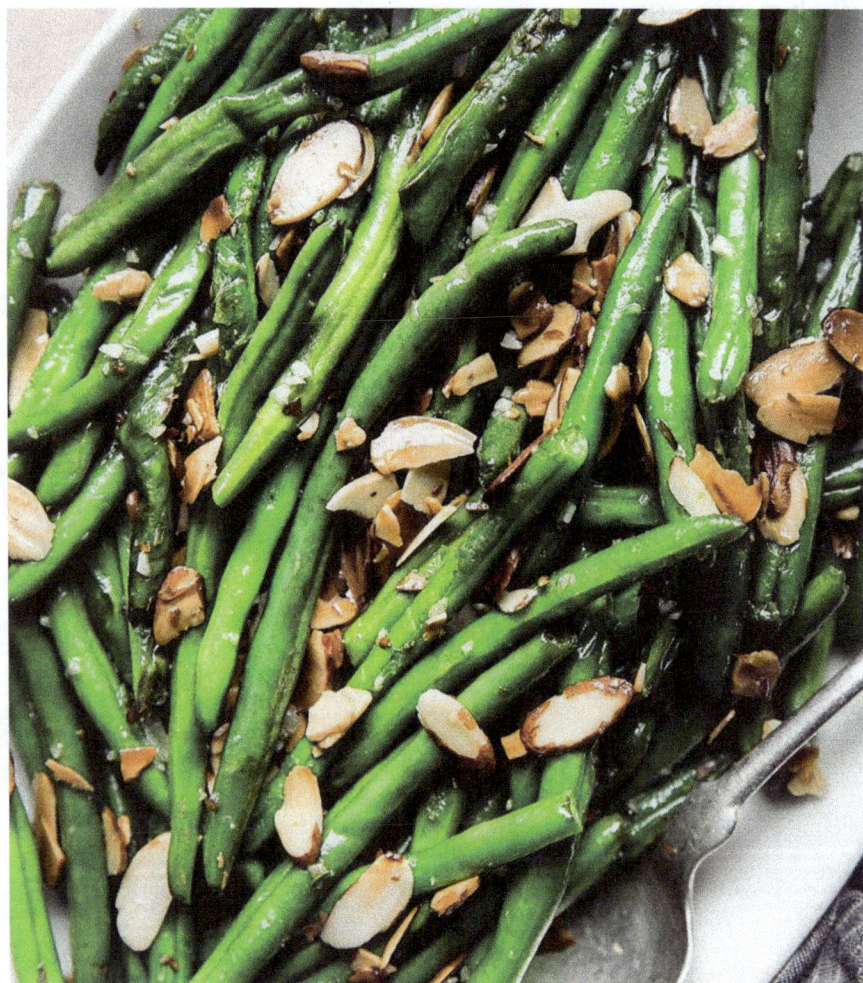

Ingredients

3–4 cups trimmed fresh green beans
2 tablespoons olive oil
1 tablespoon lemon zest
2 tablespoons lemon juice
1 teaspoon sea salt
½ cup roughly chopped toasted almonds

Directions

1. Fill the water bath with water. Set your machine temperature to 183°F/84°C.

2. Place the green beans, oil and lemon zest in a food-safe bag and vacuum seal the bag. Make sure the beans are lined up side by side and not stacked or piled. Use multiple bags if necessary.

3. Place the beans in the water bath and cook for 45–60 minutes.

4. Remove the green beans from the bag and place on a serving plate. Drizzle with lemon juice and sprinkle with salt.

5. Top with chopped almonds and serve.

15. CARROT STICKS

Cal.: 294 | Fat: 21g | Protein: 17g

Preparation Time: 9 minutes
Cooking Time: 1 hour
Servings: 4

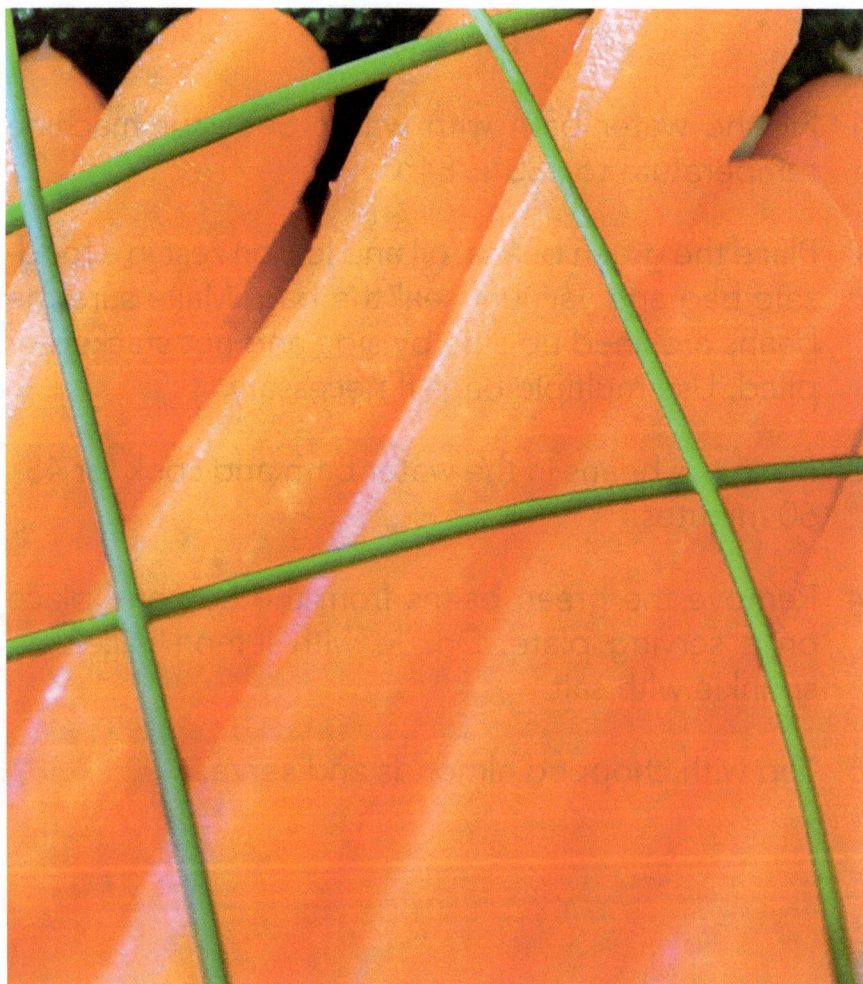

Ingredients

400 g carrots
1 tbsp. butter
1 teaspoon fennel seeds
1 teaspoon grated ginger

Directions

1. Peel finely the washed carrots with a potato peeler and cut into sticks.

2. Place these next to each other in a vacuum bag. Add the fennel seeds and ginger to the bag and close the bag airtight.

3. Preheat the water bath to 176°F/80°C and cook the carrot sticks for 60 minutes. The whole thing also works in the steamer.

4. In the end, rinse the carrots in the bag with cold, preferably ice, water. Finally, toss the carrots through hot butter in a pan.

16. TEQUILA LIME CHICKEN

Cal.: 131 | Fat: 3.4g | Protein: 12.8g

Preparation Time: 20 minutes
Cooking Time: 1 hour
Servings: 4

Ingredients

3 tablespoons olive oil
3 tablespoons tequila
1 tablespoon lime zest, from about 2 limes
4 garlic cloves, minced
1 1/4 teaspoons ancho chili powder
½ teaspoon ground coriander
1/4 teaspoon dried oregano
1 1/4 teaspoons salt
½ teaspoon freshly ground black pepper
2 teaspoons honey
4 boneless skinless chicken breasts
1 lime, sliced into wedges, for serving

Directions

1. Set your immersion circulator for 150°F/65.5°C.

2. Season the chicken with salt and pepper and set aside.

3. Combine all of the other ingredients in a bowl and stir.

4. Place the chicken breasts in a vacuum-sealed bag, add 2/3 of the seasoning mixture, and seal. The vacuum-sealed bag will marinate the meat as it cooks.

5. Place in the water bath and cook for at least 1 hour and not more than 2.

6. When you are almost finished cooking, heat your broiler to high.

7. Remove the chicken from the bag and pat dry with paper towels.

8. Place on a baking sheet and baste with the remaining seasoning mixture.

9. Cook under the broiler for just long enough for the chicken to char. Flip the chicken over and char that side.

10. Serve immediately. This dish goes well with a fresh corn salad.

17. NAPKIN DUMPLINGS

Cal.: 393 | Fat: 31g | Protein: 17g

Preparation Time: 12 minutes
Cooking Time: 75 minutes
Servings: 4

Ingredients

250 g cubes of dumpling bread
250 ml milk
½ teaspoon salt
1 handful of parsley
2 tbsp. butter
3 eggs
Some grated nutmeg

Directions

1. Put the dumpling bread in a bowl.

2. Sauté briefly the parsley in hot butter and mix with the dumpling bread.

3. Separate eggs. Mix the egg yolks with salt, milk and a little nutmeg. Mix this mixture with the dumpling bread.

4. Beat the egg whites until stiff and mix carefully with the dumpling bread.

5. Cover and let rest for ½ hour.

6. Preheat the water bath to 180°F/82°C.

7. Knead the mass quickly and shape into two rolls. The length and thickness depend on the Sous Vide pot used.

8. Seal the rolls individually or side by side in a suitable bag and cook for 60 minutes.

9. Take the dumpling rolls out of the bath and cut into slices for serving.

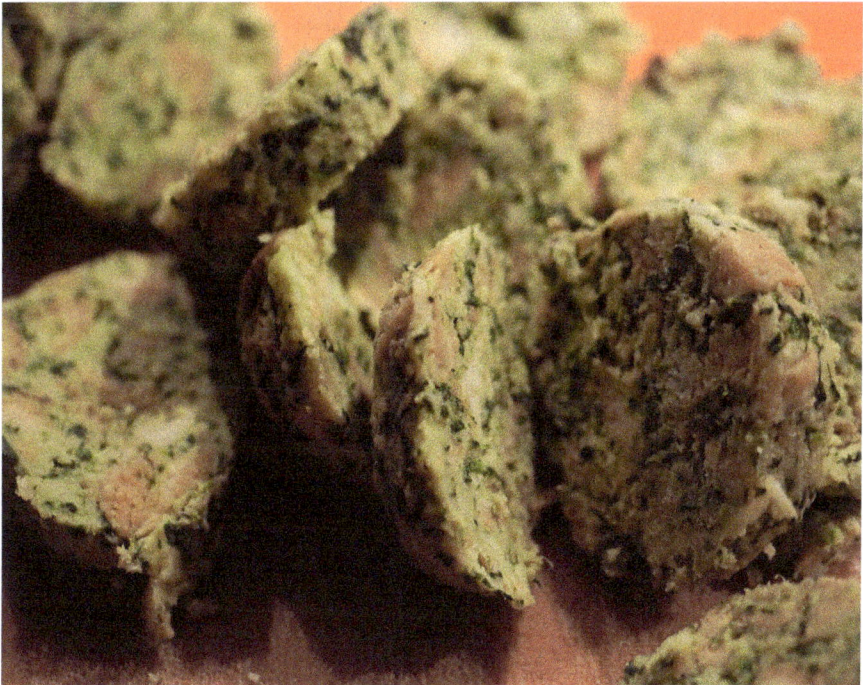

18. TURKEY WITH ARUGULA AND EGGS

Cal.: 391 | Fat: 22g | Protein: 41g

Preparation Time: 11 minutes
Cooking Time: 16 minutes
Servings: 6

Ingredients

1½ tbsp. melted butter
2 large eggs
1 pound of cooked and shredded turkey
Salt and freshly ground black pepper, to taste
3 tsp. butter
¼ cup heavy cream
2 cups of fresh baby arugula

Directions

1. Fill water in 6 ramekins.

2. Fill water halfway up the height of the ramekins.

3. Apply butter to your clean ramekins.

4. Preheat the water to 168°F/75°C.

5. Whisk 1 egg over each ramekin and add cream,

butter, black pepper and salt.

6. Place the ramekins on the baking rack and cook for 14 minutes.

7. Serve with cooked turkey.

8. Enjoy!

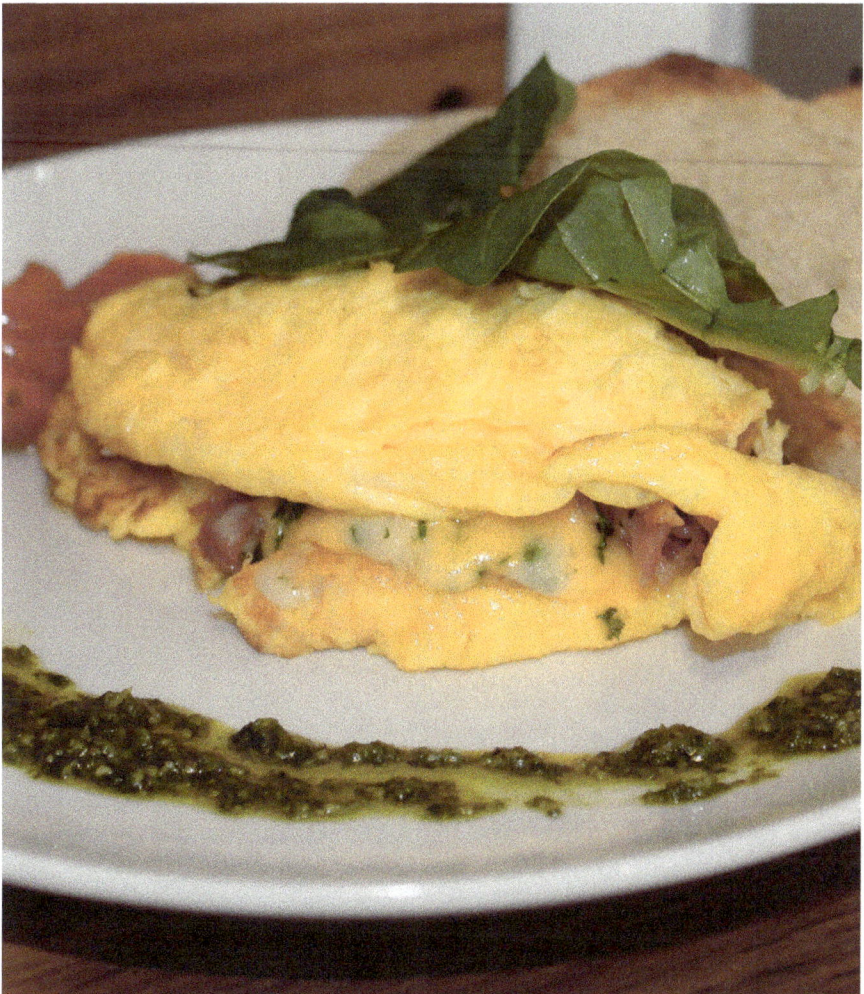

19. ROSEMARY FAVA BEANS

Cal.: 333 | Fat: 9.8g | Protein: 19.7g

Preparation Time: 11 minutes
Cooking Time: 70 minutes
Servings: 4

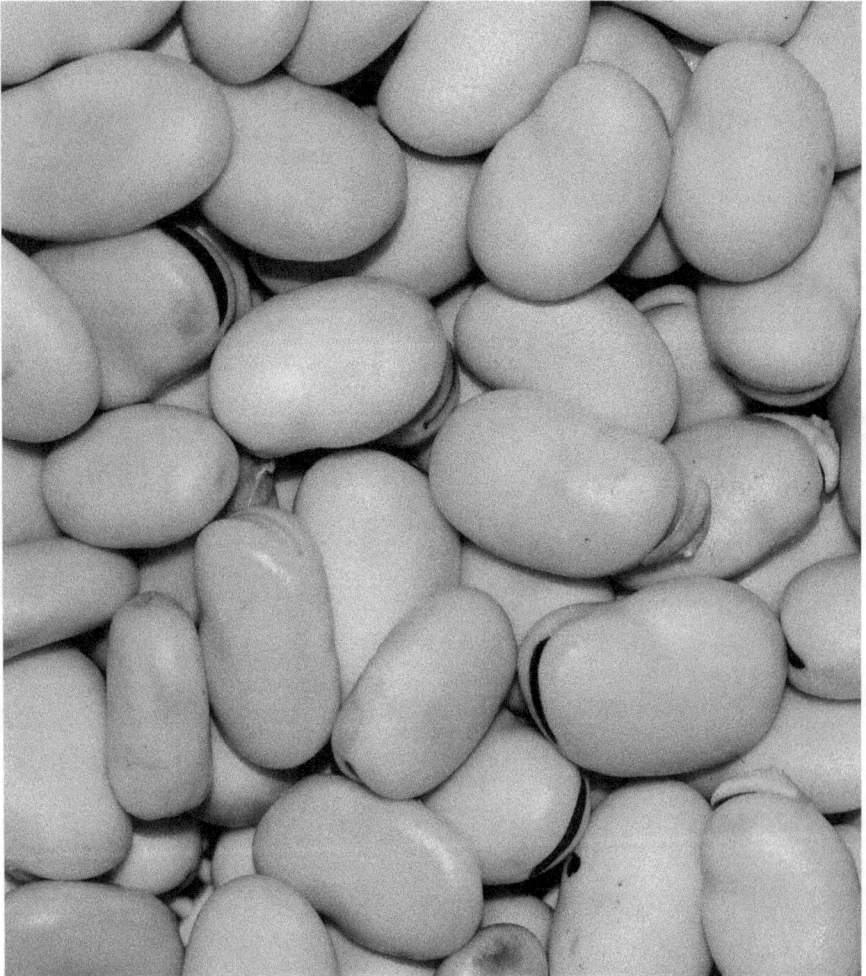

Ingredients

1.25lb. Fava beans, cleaned
½ teaspoon salt
2 sprigs rosemary
¼ teaspoon caraway seeds
1 pinch black pepper
3 tablespoons cold butter

Directions

1. Preheat the Sous Vide machine to 176°F/80°C.

2. Blanche the fava beans in simmering water for 1 minute. Drain and divide between two bags.

3. Season the beans with salt, pepper, and caraway seeds.

4. Add 1 tablespoon of butter per bag, and vacuum seals the bags.

5. Immerse the bags in water and cook for 70 minutes.

6. Remove the veggies from the bag.

7. Heat remaining butter in a skillet. Toss in the beans and coat the beans with butter.

8. Serve warm.

20. TOMATO CONFIT

Cal.: 30 | Fat: 0.3g | Protein: 1.3g

Preparation Time: 15 minutes
Cooking Time: 20 minutes
Servings: 4

Ingredients

1.25 lb. Cherry tomatoes (red, orange, yellow)
1 pinch Fleur de sel
6 black peppercorns
1 teaspoon cane sugar
2 tablespoons Bianco Aceto Balsamico
2 sprigs rosemary

Directions

1. Preheat the Sous Vide machine to 126°F/52°C.

2. Heat water in a pot and bring to a simmer.

3. Make a small incision at the bottom of each tomato.

4. Place the tomatoes into simmering water and simmer for 30 seconds.

5. Remove from the water and peel their skin.

6. Divide the tomatoes between two sous-vide bags.

7. Sprinkle the tomatoes with salt, peppercorns, sugar and Aceto Balsamico. Add 1 sprig of rosemary per bag.

8. Vacuum-seal the bags, but just to 90%. Tomatoes are soft, and they can turn into mush.

9. Immerse tomatoes in water and cook for 20 minutes.

10. Remove the tomatoes from the cooker and immerse in ice-cold water for 5 minutes.

11. Transfer the tomatoes to a bowl and serve with fresh mozzarella.

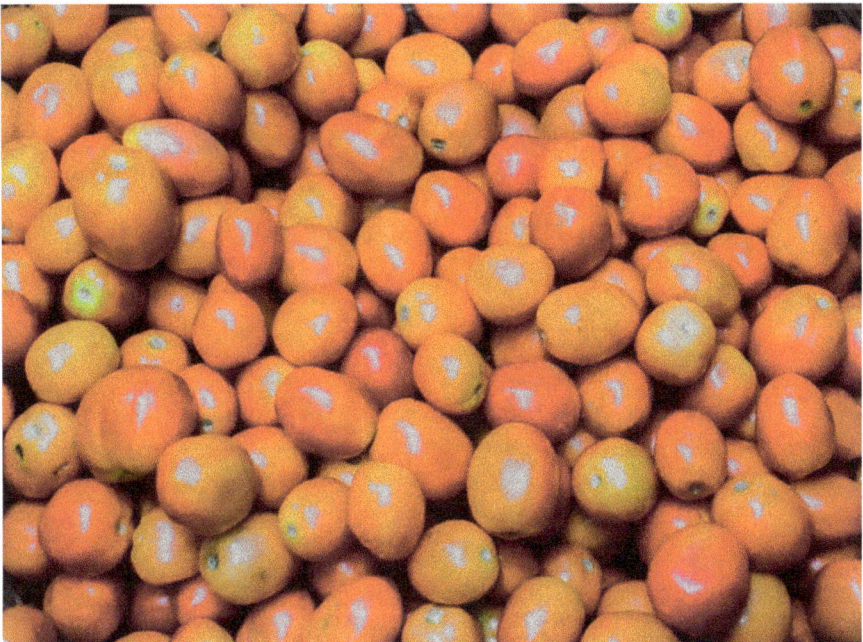

21. SMOKY SOLE FISH

Cal.: 298 | Fat: 22.9g | Protein: 22.4g

Preparation Time: 11 minutes
Cooking Time: 30 minutes
Servings: 2

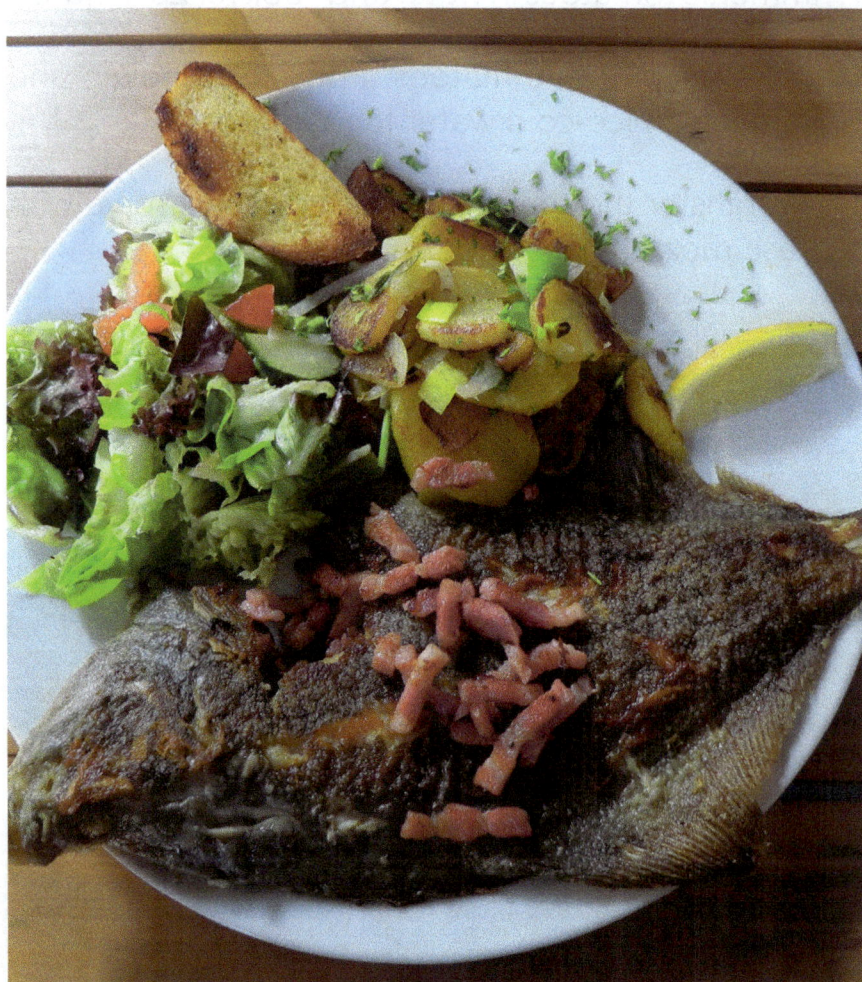

Ingredients

2 5oz. sole fish fillets
2 tablespoons olive oil
2 slices bacon
½ tablespoon lemon juice
Salt and pepper, to taste

Directions

1. Preheat the Sous Vide machine to 132°F/56°C.

2. Cook the bacon in a non-stick skillet and cook bacon until crispy.

3. Remove the bacon and place aside.

4. Season fish fillets with salt, pepper and lemon juice. Brush the fish with olive oil.

5. Place the fish in a bag. Top the fish with the bacon. Vacuum seal the bag.

6. Immerse in a water bath and cook for 25 minutes.

7. Remove the fish from the bag.

8. Serve while warm.

22. AROMATIC ROSEMARY CHICKEN

Cal.: 195 | Fat: 9.3g | Protein: 22.3g

Preparation Time: 60 minutes
Cooking Time: 2 hours
Servings: 4

Ingredients

4 chicken breasts

For the brine:
2 cups of chicken stock
4 tablespoons salt
2 tablespoons brown sugar

For the rosemary sauce:
1 stick of butter
2 teaspoons rosemary, chopped
1 teaspoon garlic powder
½ teaspoon paprika
½ teaspoon sea salt
½ teaspoon black pepper
1 tablespoon olive oil

Directions

1. Add chicken to a shallow dish with brine, cover, and refrigerate for 60 minutes.

2. Preheat the water bath to 141°F/61°C

3. Combine rosemary sauce ingredients in a mixing bowl.

4. Add chicken breasts to a vacuum bag and seal.

5. Add to the bath and cook for 2 hours.

6. Add rosemary sauce to a pan on medium-high heat and brown for 5 minutes.

7. Remove chicken from bags, coat with butter, and brown in a frying pan on medium-high, on both sides, for 2 minutes.

8. Serve drizzled with sauce and enjoy!

23. DUCK BREAST WITH AMARENA CHERRY SAUCE

Cal.: 373 | Fat: 20.9g | Protein: 35.5g

Preparation Time: 16 minutes
Cooking Time: 1 hour
Servings: 4

Ingredients

4 duck breasts
1 small jar of Amarena cherries in syrup
1 cup red wine
4 sprigs thyme
5 tablespoons butter

Directions

1. Preheat the Sous Vide machine to 145°F/63°C. Wash and dry the duck, and then cut the skin off of it. Salt and pepper the duck to taste. Place the duck in the bag with 1 tablespoon butter and 1 sprig of thyme on each breast.

2. Seal the bag, then place in the preheated container and set the timer for 1 hour.

3. Place cherries and wine in a pan and bring to a boil over high heat.

4. Reduce the temperature to medium heat and simmer until the sauce becomes thick. Take the pan off the heat.

5. When the duck is cooked, pat it dry and heat a skillet on medium heat with a tablespoon of butter.

6. Once the skillet is hot, add in the duck and sear it for about a minute per side.

7. Serve topped with the cherry sauce.

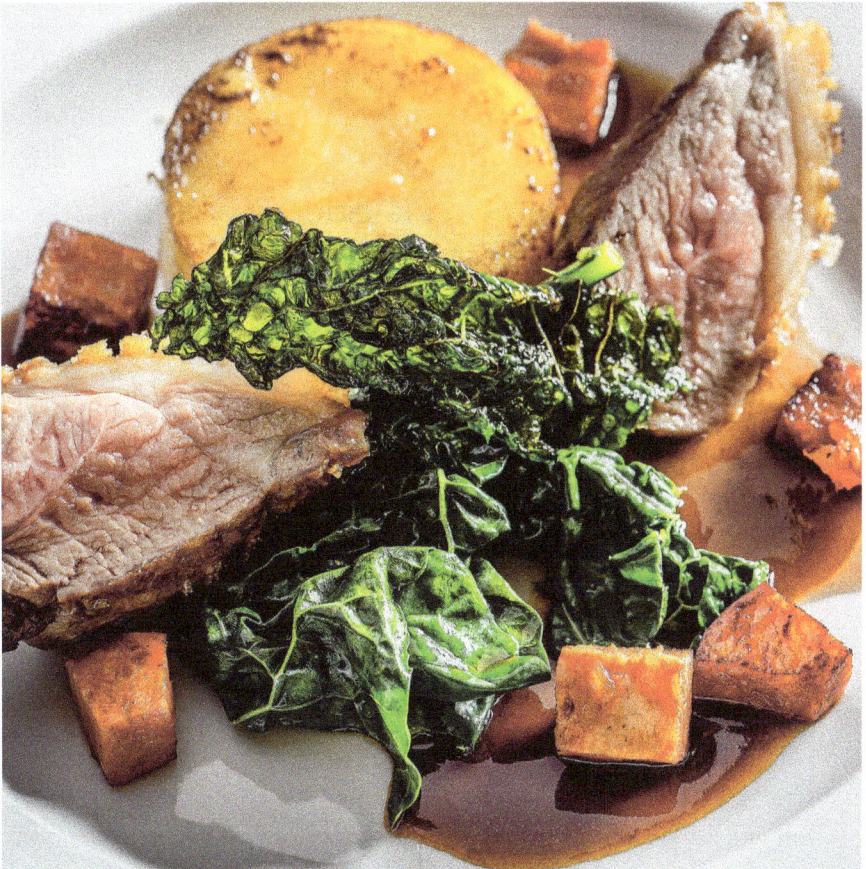

24. AMAZING HAM

Cal.: 146 | Fat: 9g | Protein: 19g

Preparation Time: 25 minutes
Cooking Time: 8 hours
Servings: 4

Ingredients

1/3 teaspoon salt
1 teaspoon chili flakes
1 teaspoon butter
1-pound ham
½ teaspoon ground black pepper
1 tablespoon apple cider vinegar
1 tablespoon honey

Directions

1. In a bowl, thoroughly mix all the ingredients except the ham and the butter.

2. Apply the vinegar mixture over the ham.

3. Transfer the ham into a Ziploc bag, remove the excess air and seal the bag.

4. Prepare your water bath to a temperature of 142°F/61°C.

5. Then transfer the sealed bag into the preheated water bath and cook for 8 minutes.

6. Once cooked, remove the cooked ham and apply butter all over it.

7. Preheat your oven to 488°F.

8. Place the cooked ham in an oven pan and cook for 10 minutes.

9. Remove the ham and shred on a platter.

10. Serve and enjoy immediately!

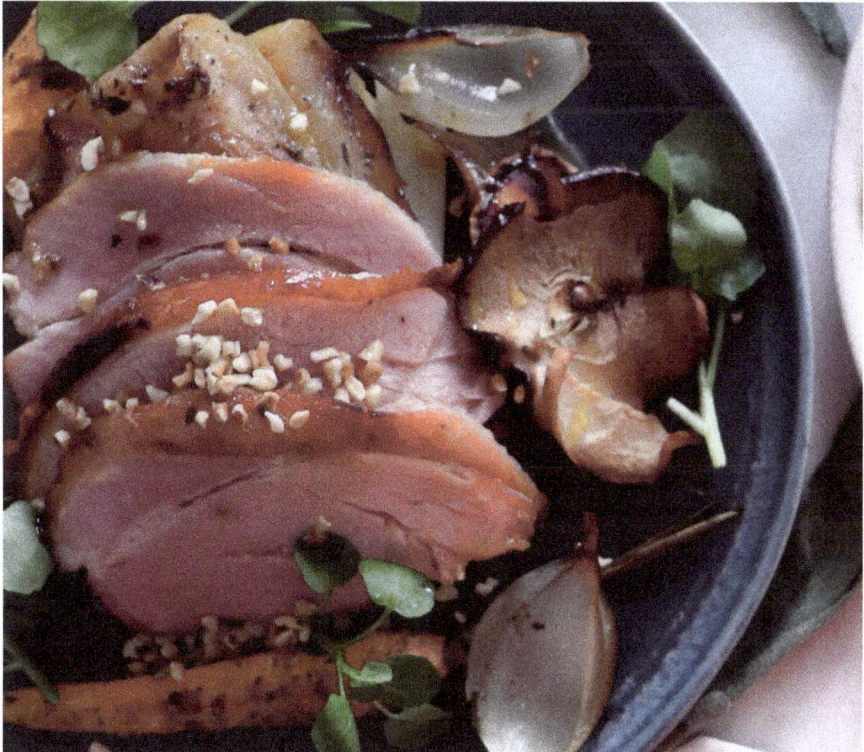

25. TANDOORI LAMB CHOPS

Cal.: 308 | Fat: 12.7g | Protein: 42.9g

Preparation Time: 1 hour
Cooking Time: 3 hours
Servings: 8

Ingredients

8 lamb rib chops (2-½ pounds)
3/4 cups Greek yogurt
1/4 cup heavy cream
3 tablespoons fresh lemon juice
1 (3-inch piece) fresh ginger, peeled and minced
4 large garlic cloves, minced
1 tablespoon malt vinegar
1 tablespoon garam masala
1 tablespoon ground cumin
1 tablespoon paprika
½ teaspoon cayenne pepper
Salt

Directions

1. Set your Sous Vide Machine to 135°F/57.2°C.

2. In a large bowl, whisk the yogurt with heavy cream, lemon juice, ginger, garlic, malt vinegar, garam masala, cumin, paprika, cayenne and 1 teaspoon salt.

3. Place lamb chops in a large vacuum-sealed bag or place two to three chops in smaller bags.

4. Pour the yogurt marinade over the lamb and seal using your vacuum-sealed.

5. Place the bag in the refrigerator to marinate for 2 hours.

6. When your water bath is ready, Immerse the bag and cook for at least 2 hours and not more than 3 hours.

7. When the lamb is almost finished, heat your oven to 450°F/230°C.

8. Remove the lamb from the bag and transfer to a baking sheet.

9. Cook in the oven for 6 minutes and turn the chops over. Cook an additional 6 minutes and serve.

26. SOFT BOILED EGGS

Cal.: 109 | Fat: 5.39g | Protein: 9.02g

Preparation Time: 11 minutes
Cooking Time: 46 minutes
Servings: 2

Ingredients

4 large eggs

Directions

1. Preheat a water bath to 63°C/145°F.

2. Use a slotted spoon to kindly place the eggs in the bath. Cook for 45 minutes.

3. When the cooking time is finished, smoothly remove the eggs from the bath (once again use a slotted spoon).

4. Serve immediately.

27. GARLIC CONFIT

Cal.: 52 | Fat: 1.1g | Protein: 2.9g

Preparation Time: 11 minutes
Cooking Time: 4 hours
Servings: 8

Ingredients

Garlic (1 cup, cloves, peeled, minced)
Olive oil (1/4 cup, extra virgin)
Salt (1 tbsp.)

Directions

1. Preheat the Sous Vide machine to 190°F/88°C.

2. Add your ingredients to a vacuum seal bag.

3. Seal and set to cook in your water bath for 4 hours.

4. To finish, transfer to an airtight container and set to refrigerate for about a month.

28. FRENCH MUSSELS

Cal.: 420 | Fat: 18g | Protein: 10g

Preparation Time: 10 minutes
Cooking Time: 10 minutes
Servings: 4

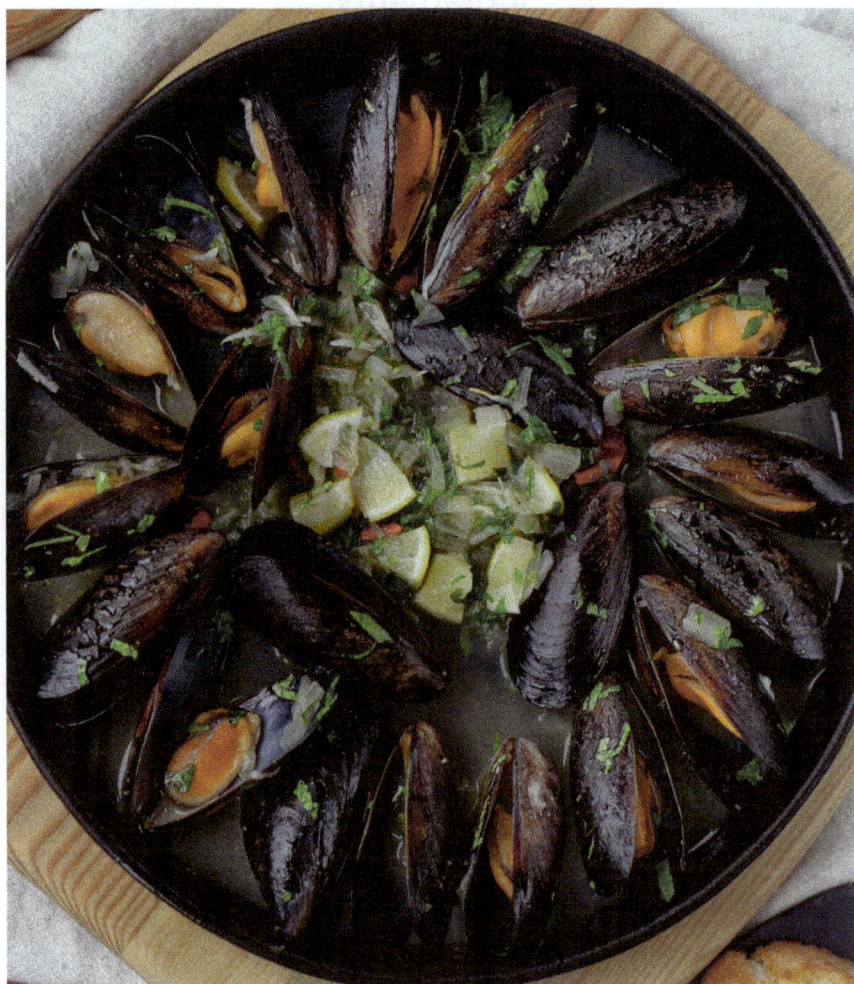

Ingredients

2 pounds mussels
1 slices fennel
4 chopped garlic cloves
2 chopped tomatoes
½ cup pastis
2 tablespoon olive oil
Salt, pepper, baguette as per need

Directions

1. Heat oil in a large saucepan. Add garlic, fennel, salt and cook for 5 minutes.

2. Add the pastis, tomatoes and simmer for 3 minutes.

3. Preheat the Sous Vide machine to 195°F/91°C.

4. Take the mussels in a large Ziploc bag and apply a vacuum to remove the air.

5. Place this bag in the water bath for 20 minutes.

6. Add the cooked mussels and cover the vessel. Cook it for 5 minutes with continuous stirring.

7. Serve hot with the baguette.

29. CHARRED CALAMARI WITH MISO AND MIRIN

Cal.: 438 | Fat: 23.2g | Protein: 19.1g

Preparation Time: 15 minutes
Cooking Time: 2 hours 30 minutes
Servings: 2

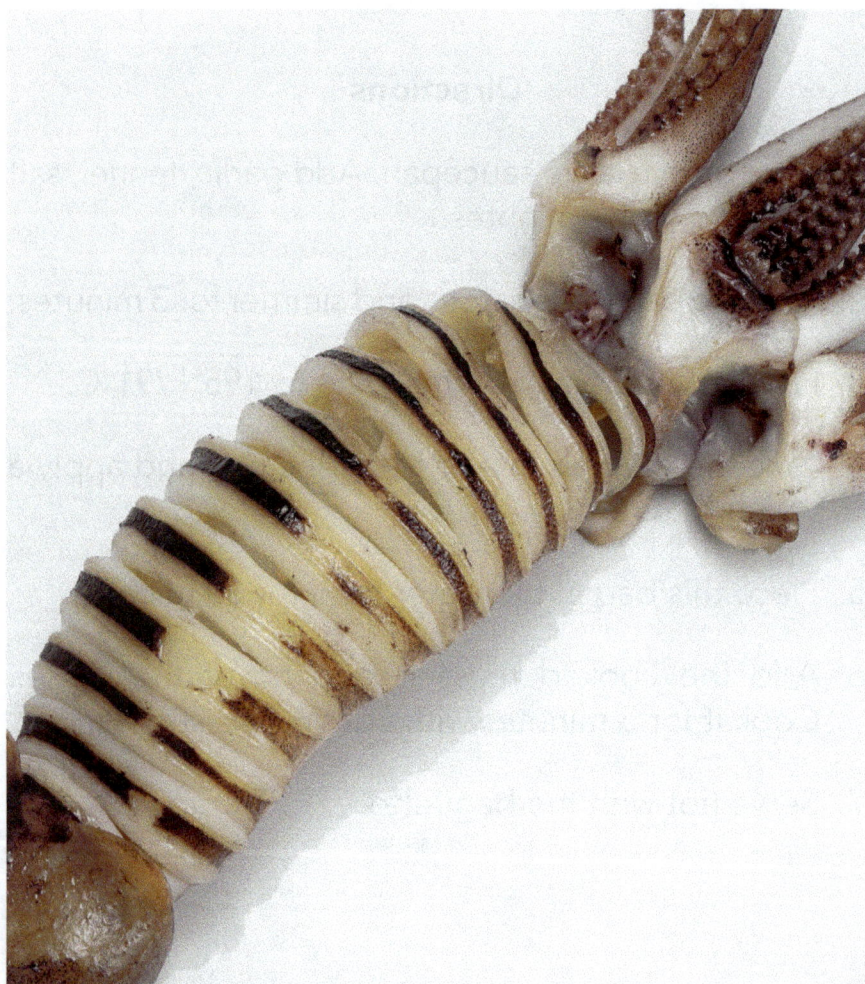

Ingredients

2 tbsp. cooking sake
2 tbsp. miso paste
2 tbsp. mirin
2 tbsp. light brown sugar
3 tbsp. chili oil
8 oz. squid bodies
1 medium lemon

Directions

1. Preheat the Sous Vide machine to 138°F/59°C. Clean and cut the calamari into thin rings and juice the lemon.

2. Mix the sake, sugar, miso and mirin in a bowl. Add in the calamari and toss until well coated. Place the calamari and marinade in the bag and cook for 2 hours.

3. In the last couple minutes of cooking, heat a grill pan on high heat.

4. When the calamari are cooked, gently pat it dry using a paper towel. Sear the calamari in batches for 30 seconds. Place seared calamari in a bowl. Mix in the lemon juice and the chili oil.

5. Serve immediately.

30. EASY MIXED VEGETABLE SOUP

Cal.: 150 | Fat: 0.3g | Protein: 1.2g

Preparation Time: 10 minutes
Cooking Time: 40 minutes
Servings: 3

Ingredients

1 sweet onion, sliced
1 tsp. garlic powder
2 cups zucchini, cut in small dices
3 oz. parmesan rind
2 cups baby spinach
2 tbsp. olive oil
1 tsp. red pepper flakes
2 cups vegetable stock
1 sprig rosemary
Salt to taste

Directions

1. Make a water bath, place a cooker in it, and set it at 185°F/85°C.

2. Toss all the ingredients with olive oil, except the garlic and salt, and place them in a vacuum-sealable bag.

3. Release air by water displacement method, seal and Immerse the bag in the water bath. Set the timer for 30 minutes.

4. Once the timer has stopped, remove and unseal the bag. Discard the rosemary. Pour the remaining ingredients into a pot and add the salt and garlic powder.

5. Once the timer has stopped, remove and unseal the bag. Discard the rosemary. Pour the remaining ingredients into a pot and add the salt and garlic powder.

6. Put the pot over medium heat and simmer for 10 minutes. Serve as a light dish.

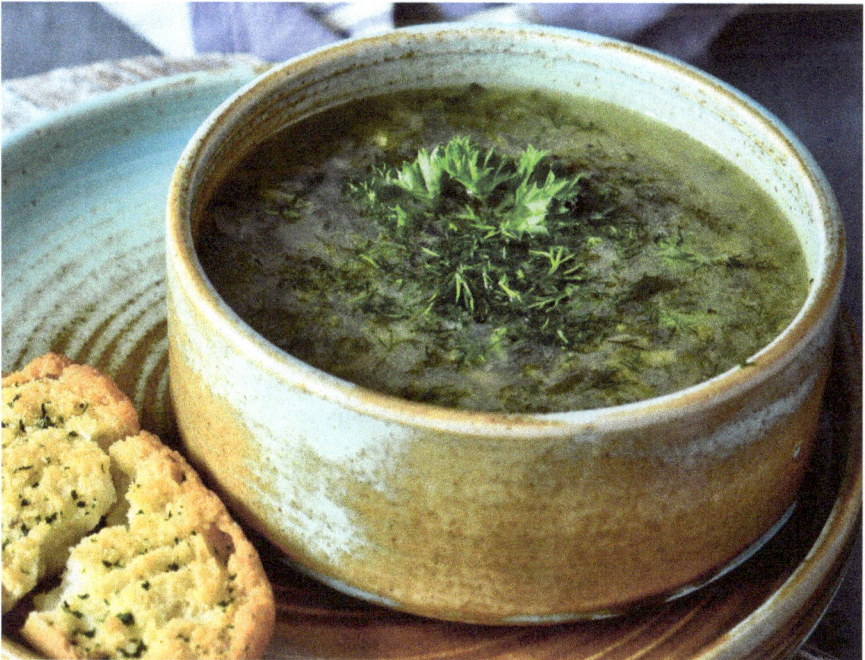

31. TENDER GARLIC ASPARAGUS

Cal.: 50 | Fat: 2.5g | Protein: 2.8g

Preparation Time: 6 minutes
Cooking Time: 1 hour
Servings: 4

Ingredients

1 lb. asparagus, cleaned and dried with a paper towel
2 teaspoons olive oil
1 tablespoon garlic powder
1 teaspoon sea salt

Directions

1. Preheat the Sous Vide machine to 135°F/57°C.

2. Toss asparagus with all ingredients until well-coated in a large mixing bowl.

3. Place asparagus, lined flat, in a vacuum sealable bag and vacuum airtight.

4. Cook for 1 hour.

5. Serve immediately with your favorite dish.

---

32. LEMON AND PARMESAN BROCCOLI

Cal.: 63 | Fat: 4.8g | Protein: 1.7g

Preparation Time: 11 minutes
Cooking Time: 52 minutes
Servings: 5

Ingredients

1 head of broccoli
2 tablespoons butter
Salt and pepper
Parmesan cheese, for sprinkling
1 lemon

Directions

1. Preheat the Sous Vide machine to 185°F/85°C. Cut the head of broccoli into large pieces.

2. Put the broccoli and butter in a bag. Salt and pepper to taste.

3. Place the bag in your preheated container and set your timer for 45 minutes.

4. Transfer broccoli to a plate and add the lemon juice and top with cheese to serve.

33. PAPRIKA BELL PEPPER PURÉE

Cal.: 20 | Fat: 0.2g | Protein: 0.9g

Preparation Time: 20 minutes
Cooking Time: 2 hours 23 minutes
Servings: 4

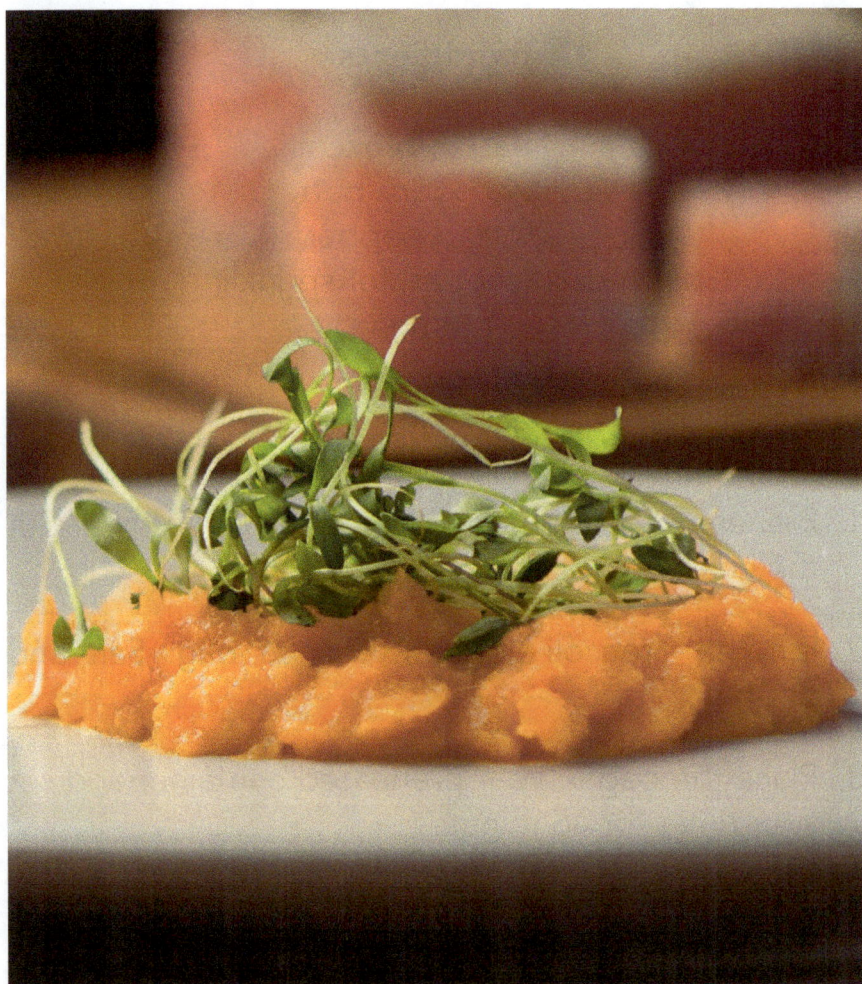

Ingredients

8 Red Bell Peppers, cored
1/3 cup Olive Oil
2 tbsp. Lemon Juice
3 garlic cloves, crushed
2 tsp. Sweet Paprika

Directions

1. Make a water bath and place a cooker in it and set it at 183°F/84°C.

2. Put the bell peppers, garlic, and olive oil in a vacuum-sealable bag.

3. Release air by the water displacement method, seal and Immerse the bags in the water bath. Set the timer for 20 minutes and cook.

4. Once the timer has stopped, remove the bag and unseal it. Transfer the bell pepper and garlic to a blender and purée to smooth.

5. Place a pan over medium heat; add bell pepper purée and the remaining listed ingredients. Cook for 3 minutes. Serve warm or cold as a dip.

34. PICKLED ASPARAGUS

Cal.: 145 | Fat: 19g | Protein: 10g

Preparation Time: 21 minutes
Cooking Time: 30 minutes
Servings: 4

Ingredients

12 oz. asparagus, woody ends trimmed
2/3 cup white wine vinegar
2/3 cup water
3 tbsp. sugar
1 tbsp. sea salt
½ tsp. whole peppercorns
½ tsp. yellow or brown mustard seeds
¼ tsp. coriander seeds
2 garlic cloves, peeled and sliced in half lengthwise
1 bay leaf
Fresh chili pepper, sliced in half

Directions

1. Preheat the Sous Vide machine to 190°F/87.8°C.

2. Place everything but the asparagus in a small pot and heat on high heat until it boils. Carefully stir the mixture until the sugar dissolves.

3. Place the asparagus in a single layer row in the bag(s) you're going to use to sous, along with the heated mixture and seal the bag.

4. Place the bag in your preheated water and set the timer for 10 min.

5. While asparagus is cooking, prepare an ice bath (half ice half water).

6. Place the cooked asparagus, still in the bag in the ice bath and let it chill for 15 minutes before serving.

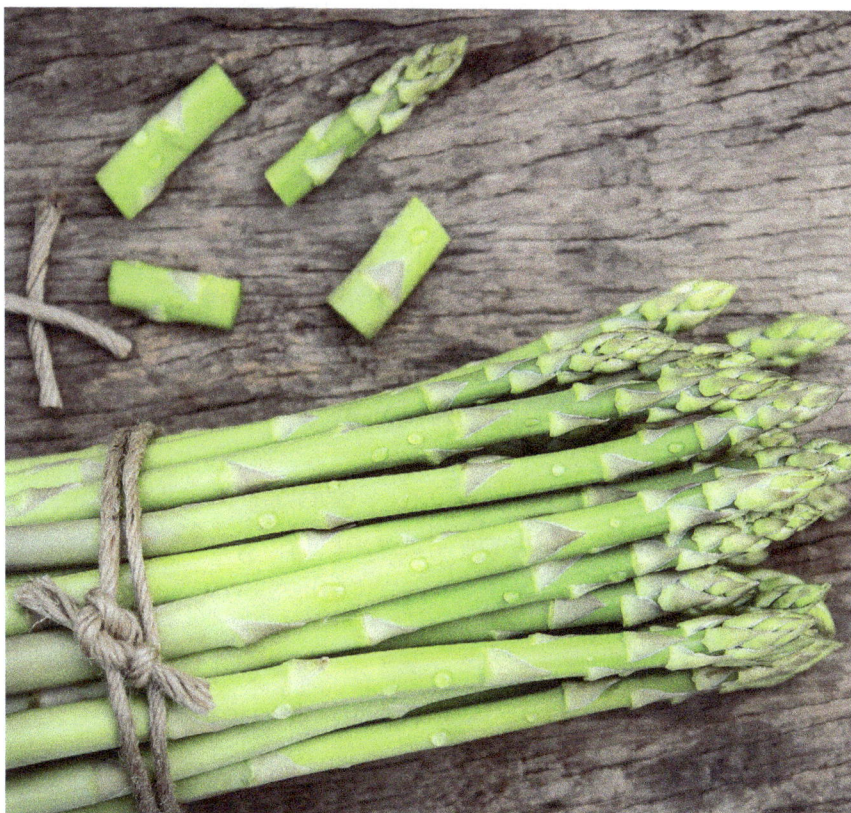

35. ARTICHOKE HEARTS WITH GREEN CHILIES

Cal.: 47 | Fat: 0.2g | Protein: 3.3g

Preparation Time: 1 hour 15 minutes
Cooking Time: 33 minutes
Servings: 6

Ingredients

2 onions, quartered
3 garlic cloves, minced
15 oz. artichoke hearts, soaked for 1 hour, drained and chopped
18 oz. frozen spinach, thawed
5 oz. green chilies
3 tbsp. olive oil mayonnaise
3 tbsp. whipped cream cheese

Directions

1. Make a water bath, place a cooker in it, and set it at 181°F/82°C. Divide the onions, garlic, artichoke hearts, spinach and green chilies into 2 vacuum-sealable bags.

2. Release air by the water displacement method, seal and Immerse the bags in the water bath. Set the timer for 30 minutes to cook.

3. Once the timer has stopped, remove and unseal the bag. Purée the ingredients using a blender. Place a pan over medium heat and add the butter.

4. Once it has melted, add the vegetable purée, lemon juice, olive oil mayonnaise, and cream cheese. Season with salt and pepper. Stir and cook for 3 minutes. Serve warm with a side of vegetable strips.

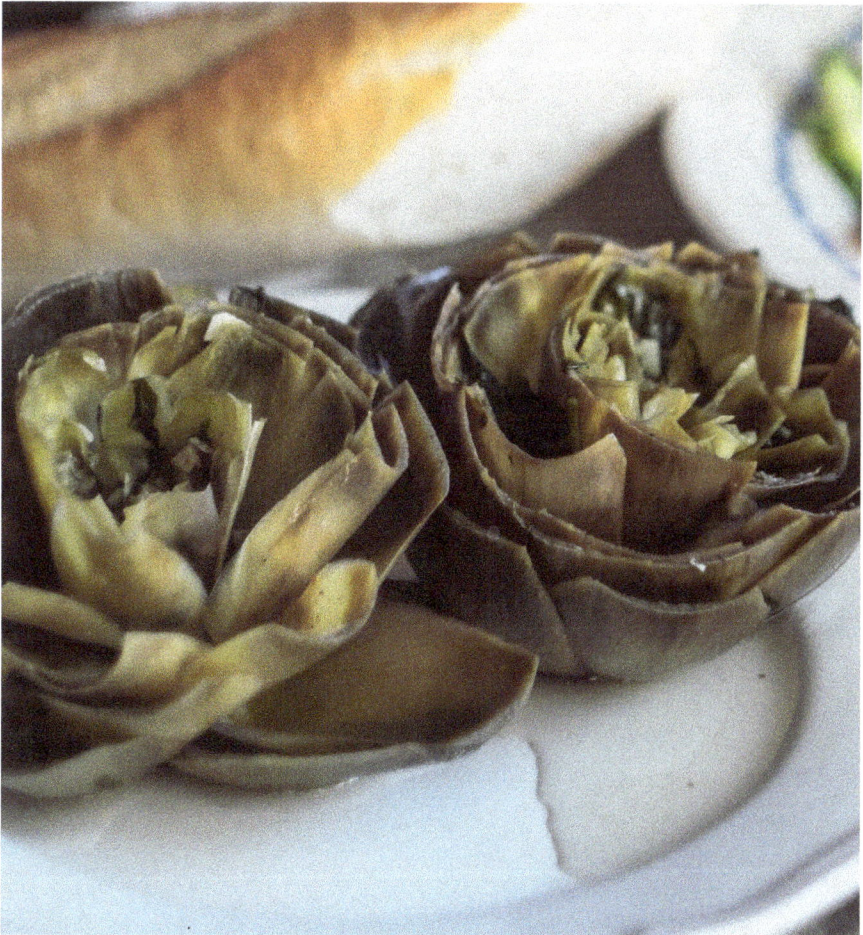

36. SQUASH AND LENTIL STEW

Cal.: 325 | Fat: 19g | Protein: 4g

Preparation Time: 15 minutes
Cooking Time: 24 hours 35 minutes
Servings: 6

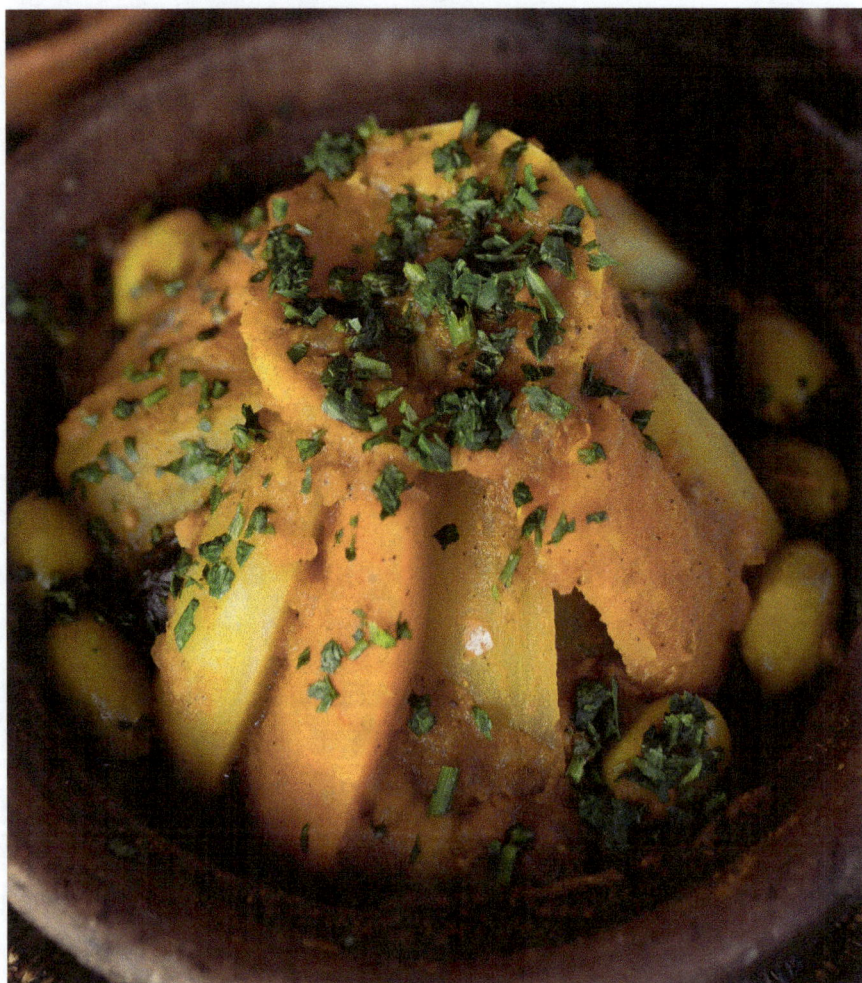

Ingredients

1 pound green lentils
2 sliced shallots
1 butternut squash
Cups baby spinach
Cups vegetable broth
1 tablespoon chopped ginger
1 teaspoon coriander powder
½ teaspoon cardamom powder
1 tablespoon vinegar
Salt and pepper

Directions

1. Take the squash and peel it. Cut it into 1 ½" pieces.

2. Preheat the Sous Vide machine to 165°F/74°C.

3. Take the lentils, squash in the bag.

4. Place the bag in and cook for 5 minutes.

5. Transfer it to a cooking pan. Add shallot, ginger, oil, cardamom powder, coriander powder, salt and vegetable broth.

6. Cook on high flame for 12 minutes.

7. Add spinach, vinegar, salt, pepper and serve hot.

37. SMOKED SALMON EGGS BENEDICT

Cal.: 604 | Fat: 49g | Protein: 26.1g

Preparation Time: 8 minutes
Cooking Time: 2 hours 30 minutes
Servings: 4

Ingredients

4 eggs
8 ounces smoked salmon
2 English muffins, split
Hollandaise sauce, bagged and uncooked

Directions

1. Preheat the bath to 147°F/64°C.

2. Seal the eggs in a bag. Place the bag of eggs, and the bag of hollandaise into the bath. Cook for 2 hours.

3. 30 minutes before the end of cooking time, toast and butter the English muffins.

4. Remove eggs and sauce from the bath.

5. Pour sauce into a blender and blend until smooth

and meanwhile, cold eggs in a bowl of cold water.

6. Arrange 2 ounces of smoked salmon on each English muffin half to form a cup that will hold the poached egg.

7. Carefully crack each egg over a slotted spoon held over a bowl to allow the excess white to drip away.

8. Place one egg in each smoked salmon cup.

9. Top with hollandaise sauce.

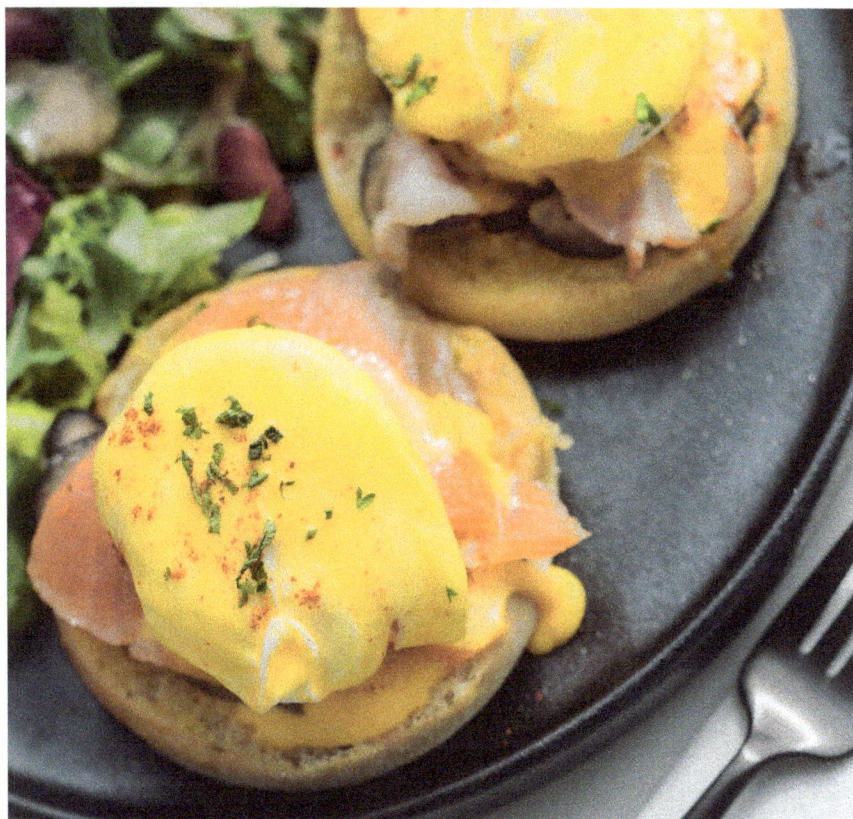

38. CARAMELIZED YOGURT WITH GRILLED BERRIES

Cal.: 101 | Fat: 3.5g | Protein: 5.4g

Preparation Time: 60 minutes
Cooking Time: 12 hours
Servings: 8

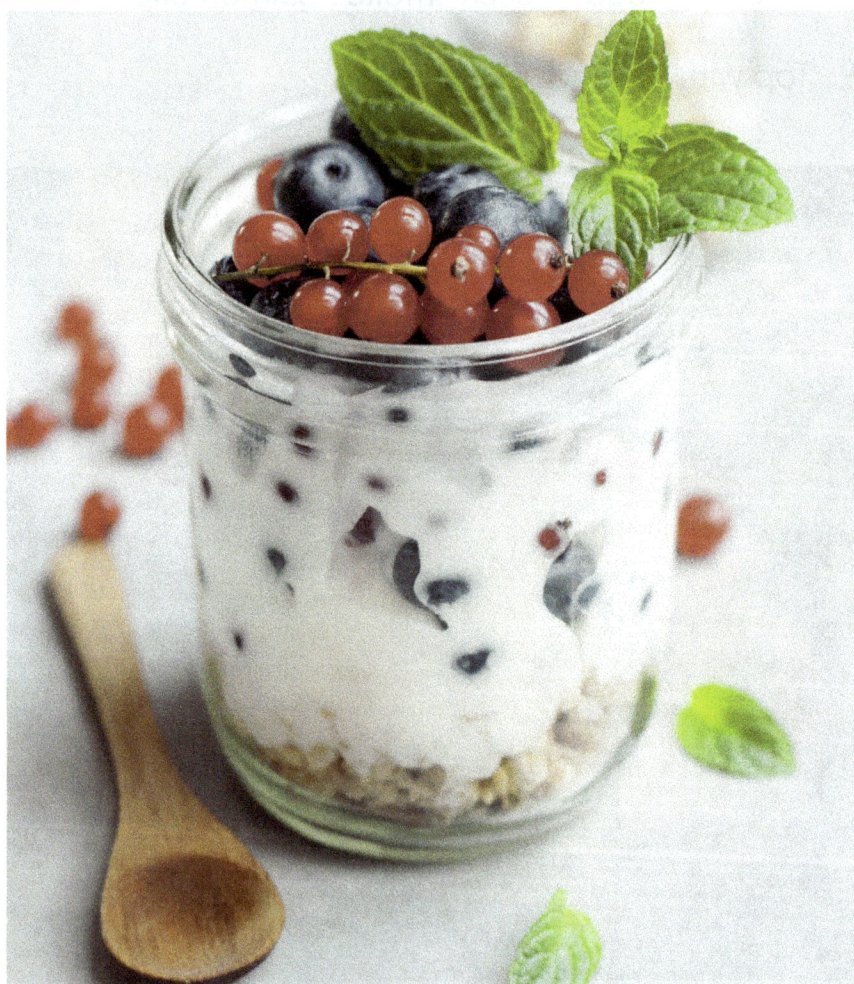

Ingredients

1 lb. natural yogurt plus 3.5 oz. natural yogurt
12 oz. blueberries
12 oz. raspberries
Mint for garnish

Directions

1. Preheat your Sous Vide Machine to 162°F/72°C.

2. Place the yogurt in a bag and place the bag in the preheated container and set your timer for 12 hours.

3. When nearly finished cooking, prepare an ice bath.

4. Once cooked, place the bag in a bowl, and put the bowl in the ice bath. Allow the yogurt to cool.

5. Open the bag and pour the yogurt into a colander or sieve that's lined with the muslin cloth. Position the sieve over a bowl and let strain for about an hour.

6. Slowly whisk in the 3.5 ounces of yogurt. Grill the berries on a very hot grill for a short time or heat with a kitchen torch. Garnish with mint to serve.

39. APPLE COBBLER

Cal.: 170 | Fat: 2.4g | Protein: 2g

Preparation Time: 9 minutes
Cooking Time: 3 hours 40 minutes
Servings: 6

Ingredients

1 cup milk
2 green apples, cubed
1 tsp. butter
7 tbsp. flour
4 tbsp. brown sugar
1 tsp. ground Cardamom

Directions

1. Preheat the Sous Vide machine to 190°F/88°C. Whisk together the butter, sugar, milk and cardamom. Stir in the flour gradually. Fold in the apples. Divide the mixture between 6 small jars. Seal the jars and place them in the water bath. Cook for 3 ½ hours.

40. BLUEBERRY AND LEMON COMPOTE

Cal.: 181 | Fat: 1g | Protein: 1g

Preparation Time: 11 minutes
Cooking Time: 1 hour
Servings: 4

Ingredients

½ cup ultrafine sugar
1 tablespoon freshly squeezed lemon juice
1 tablespoon lemon zest
1 tablespoon cornstarch
1 pound blueberries

Directions

1. Prepare your water bath by dipping the immersion circulator and increasing the temperature to 180°F/82°C. Take a medium-sized bowl and whisk in sugar, lemon zest, lemon juice and cornstarch. Mix well and add blueberries, toss to coat the berries. Transfer the whole to a zip bag and seal using the immersion method.

2. Cook for 1 hour. Remove the bag and transfer to your serving dish. Enjoy!

41. CARROT MUFFINS

Cal.: 173 | Fat: 4g | Protein: 12g

Preparation Time: 11 minutes
Cooking Time: 3 hours 20 minutes
Servings: 10

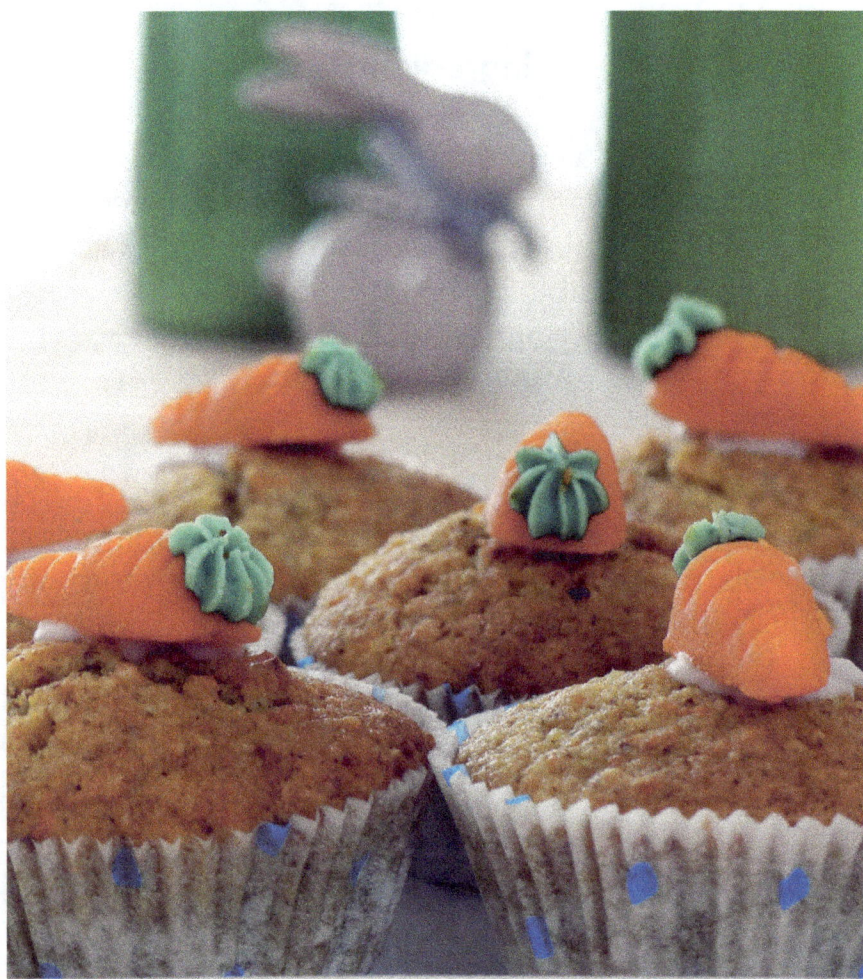

Ingredients

1 cup Flour
3 Eggs
½ cup Butter
¼ cup Heavy Cream
2 Carrots, grated
1 tsp. Lemon Juice
1 tbsp. Coconut Flour
¼ tsp. Salt
½ tsp. Baking Soda

Directions

1. Whisk the wet ingredients in one bowl and combine the dry ones in another.

2. Gently combine the 2 mixtures together.

3. Preheat the Sous Vide machine to 195°F/91°C.

4. Divide the mixture between 5 mason jars (do not fill more than halfway. Use more jars if needed).

5. Seal and immerse in the water. Cook for 3 hours. Cut into halves and serve.

42. KEY LIME PIE

Cal.: 213 | Fat: 8g | Protein: 22g

Preparation Time: 7 minutes
Cooking Time: 1 hour
Servings: 6

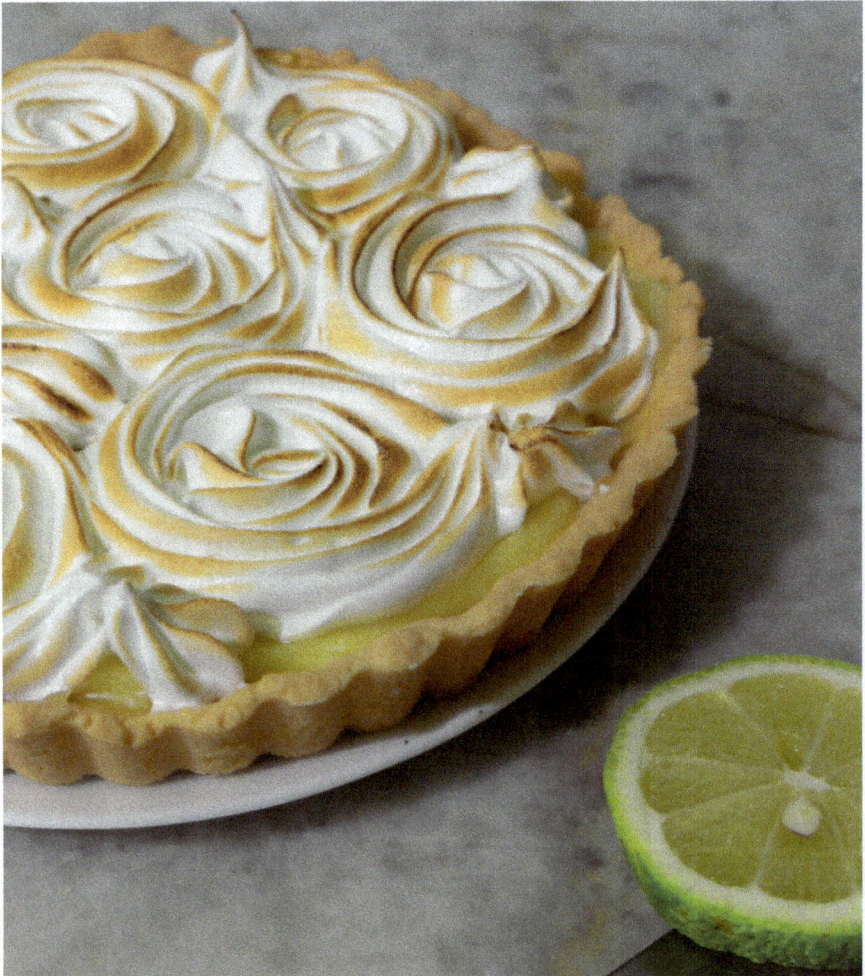

Ingredients

½ cup key lime juice
14 ounces of sweetened condensed milk
A pinch of kosher salt
6 large egg yolks
3 cups of whipped cream
1 baked graham cracker crust
1 tbsp. key lime zest

Directions

1. Preheat the Sous Vide machine to 180°F/82°C. In a blender, add in the salt, egg yolks, lime juice and condensed milk. Blend for 30 seconds or until frothy and smooth. Transfer the mixture into a Ziploc bag and seal using the water immersion method.

2. Place the Ziploc bag into the water bath. Cook in the cooker for 30 minutes. While cooking, make sure to agitate the bag several times to prevent clumps from forming.

3. Once done, remove the bag from the water bath and place on a bowl with water and ice. Once the mixture has cooled down, remove from the bag and pour into the crust.

4. Top with whipped cream and garnish with lime zest. Place in the refrigerator to chill for at least 30 minutes then serve.

43. POACHED PEARS

Cal.: 273 | Fat: 8g | Protein: 12g

Preparation Time: 11 minutes
Cooking Time: 3 hours 30 minutes
Servings: 4

Ingredients

4 ounces of gorgonzola cheese, softened
2 firm and ripe pears, peeled and cored then halved
½ cup tawny port
½ cup dried cherries, chopped
1 tsp. pure vanilla extract
2 tsp. honey
4 sprigs of mint for garnish
½ cup toasted pecans, chopped then lightly toasted

Directions

1. Preheat the Sous Vide machine to 165°F/74°C.

2. Combine the dried cherries and cheese in a bowl. Take half of the mixture and use it to fill the cavity of each half of the pear. Set the remaining mixture aside.

3. In another bowl, combine the vanilla, honey and port. Place ½ of a pear into each ramekin then

divide the sauce equally among the ramekins.

4. Place each ramekin in a Ziploc bag and seal using the water immersion method.

5. Place the bags into the water bath and cook in the cooker for 3 ½ hours. Once finished, remove the ramekins from the bags.

6. Make the remaining cherry mixture into balls. To serve, top each ramekin with the cherry cheese balls and pecans. Use the mint sprigs for garnish.

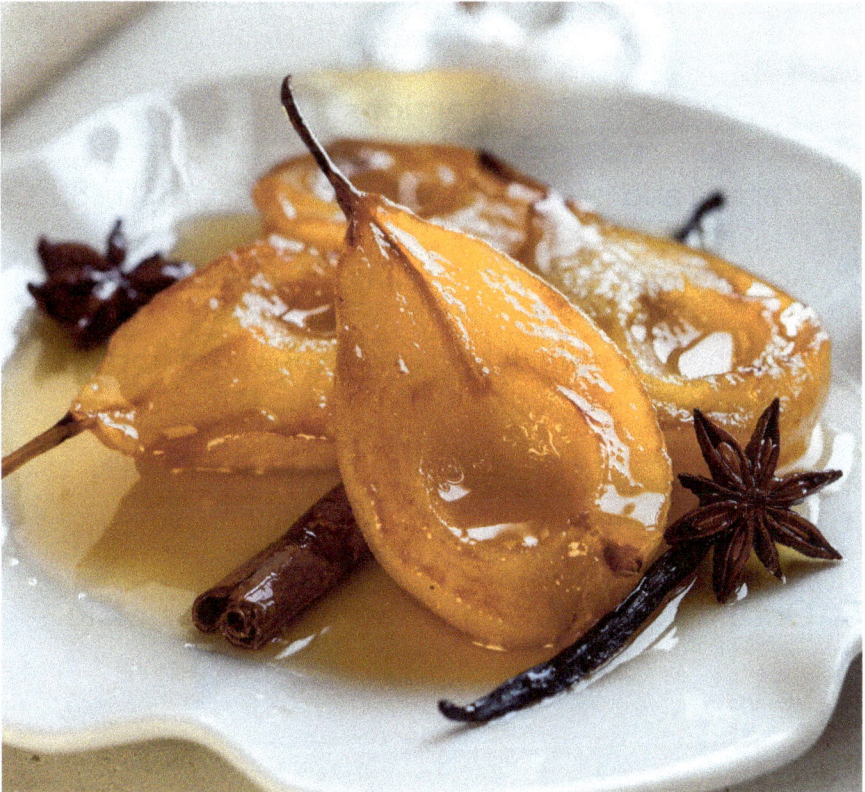

44. STRAWBERRY WATERMELON

Cal.: 33 | Fat: 0.1g | Protein: 0.2g

Preparation Time: 15 minutes
Cooking Time: 30 minutes
Servings: 1

Ingredients

1/4 cup strawberry vodka
1/4 watermelon, peeled and cubed

Directions

1. Prepare and preheat the water bath at 185°F/85°C.

2. Add watermelon and vodka to a zipper-lock bag.

3. Seal the zipper-lock bag using the water immersion method.

4. Place the sealed bag in the bath and cook for 30 minutes.

5. Once done, transfer the watermelon to a plate.

6. Serve.

45. FINGERLING POTATOES WITH ROSEMARY

Cal.: 85 | Fat: 2.7g | Protein: 1.8g

Preparation Time: 10 minutes
Cooking Time: 2 hours
Servings: 12

Ingredients

2 tablespoons olive oil
4 garlic cloves, peeled
1 sprig fresh rosemary, chopped
12 fingerling potatoes, washed
Salt, to taste
Black pepper, to taste

Directions

1. Prepare and preheat the water bath at 194°F/90°C.

2. Add potatoes and all the ingredients to a zipper-lock bag. Seal the zipper-lock bag using the water immersion method. Place the sealed bag in the bath and cook for 2 hours.

3. Once done, transfer the potatoes along with the sauce to a plate. Serve.

46. BLACKBERRY HIBISCUS DELIGHT

Cal.: 149 | Fat: 0.6g | Protein: 1.6g

Preparation Time: 11 minutes
Cooking Time: 90 minutes
Servings: 4

Ingredients

1lb. fresh blackberries
½ cup red wine vinegar
½ cup caster sugar
2 teaspoons crushed hibiscus flowers
3 bay leaves

Directions

1. Preheat the Sous Vide machine to 140°F/60°C.

2. In a saucepot, combine red wine vinegar, caster sugar, hibiscus, and bay leaves.

3. Heat until the sugar is dissolved. Allow cooling.

4. Place the blackberries and cooled syrup in a bag.

5. Vacuum seal and immerse in water.

6. Cook for 1 hour 30 minutes.

7. Remove the bag from the cooker and place in ice-cold water for 10 minutes.

8. Open carefully and transfer the content to a bowl.

9. Serve.

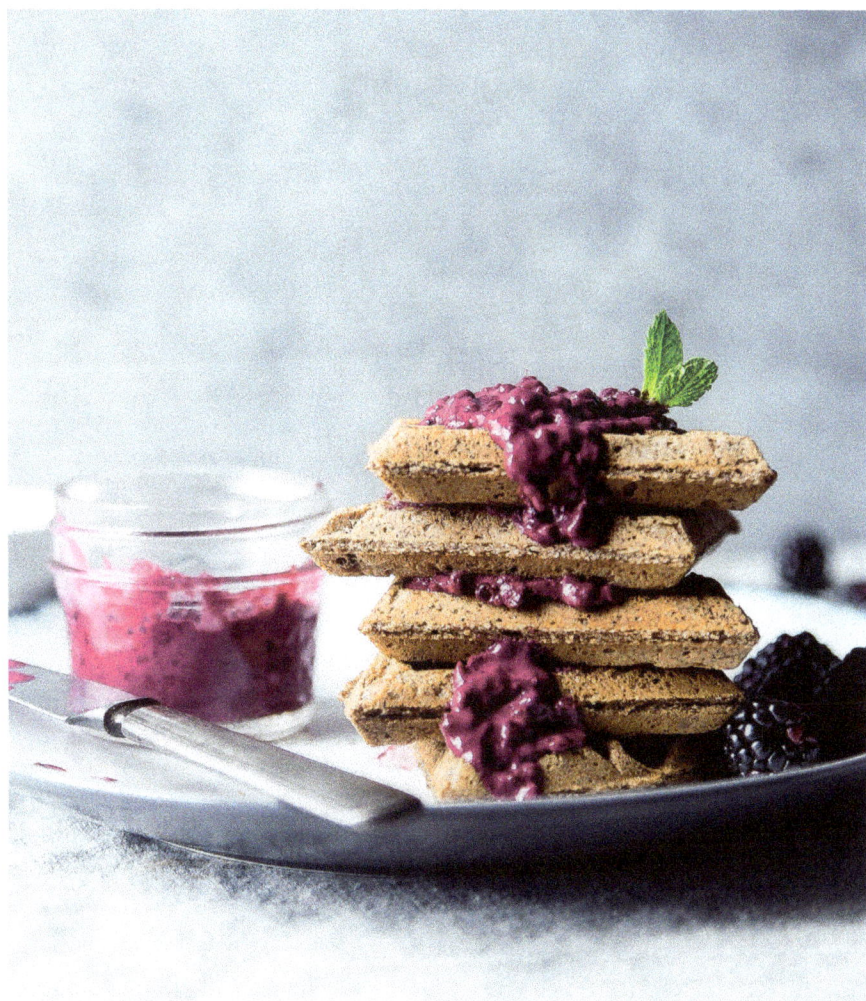

47. APRICOT AND CRANBERRY PIE

Cal.: 272 | Fat: 3g | Protein: 16g

Preparation Time: 11 minutes
Cooking Time: 2 hours 20 minutes
Servings: 4

Ingredients

2 pounds ripe apricots, bone removed, halved
½ pound cranberries
3/4 cup sugar
2 tbsp. cornstarch
2 tbsp. butter
2 tsp. ground cinnamon
1 pack puff pastry
2 tbsp. milk
2 tbsp. sugar

Directions

1. Preheat the water bath to 160°F/71°C.

2. Put the apricots, cornstarch, cranberries, sugar, cinnamon and butter in the vacuum bag and set the cooking time for 1 hour 30 minutes.

3. When the time is up, cool down the filling to the

room temperature.

4. In the meantime, preheat the oven to 375°F/190°C, grease a baking pan, and roll out 1 sheet of the pastry.

5. Pour the filling over the sheet, and cover it with another sheet, seal the sheets on the edges with your fingers.

6. Bake in the preheated oven for 35 minutes.

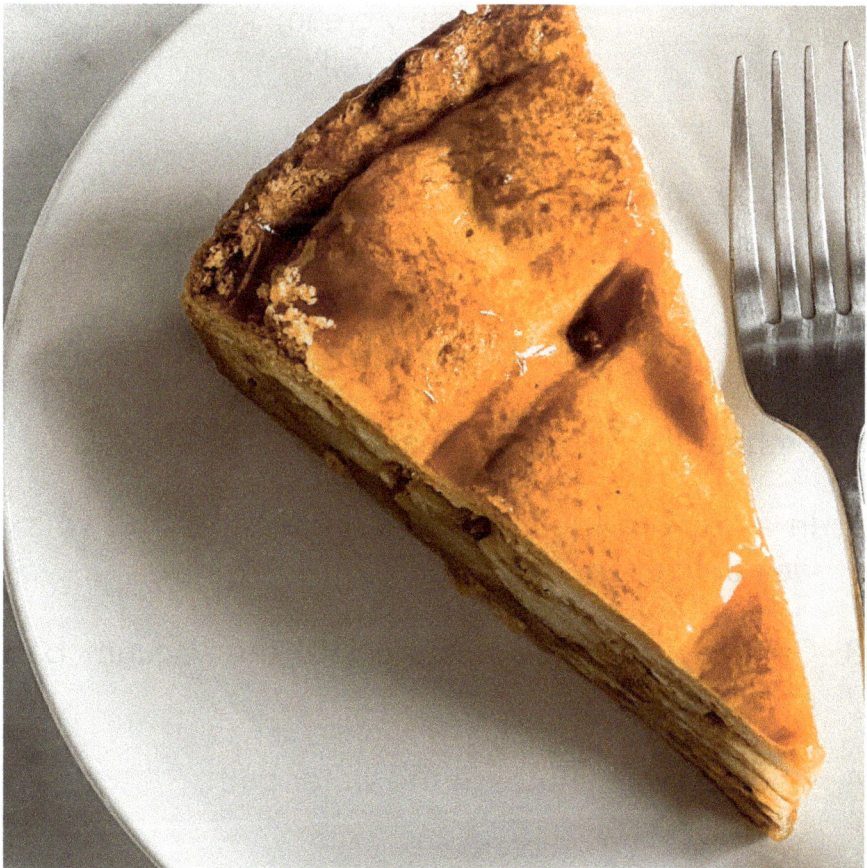

48. TANGERINE ICE CREAM

Cal.: 144 | Fat: 3g | Protein: 8g

Preparation Time: 11 minutes
Cooking Time: 24 hours 30 minutes
Servings: 6

Ingredients

1 cup mandarin (only juice and pulp)
2 cups heavy cream
6 fresh egg yolks
½ cup milk
½ cup white sugar
1/4 cup sweet condensed milk
A pinch of salt

Directions

1. Preheat the Sous Vide machine to 185°F/85°C

2. In a big bowl, combine all ingredients and whisk well until even.

3. Carefully pour the mixture into the vacuum bag and seal it.

4. Cook for 30 minutes in the water bath.

---

5. When the time is up, quick chill the vacuum bag without opening it. To do this, put it into a big bowl or container, filled with ice and water.

6. Refrigerate the vacuum bag with ice-cream for 24 hours.

7. Carefully transfer the mixture to an ice-cream machine and cook according to the instructions.

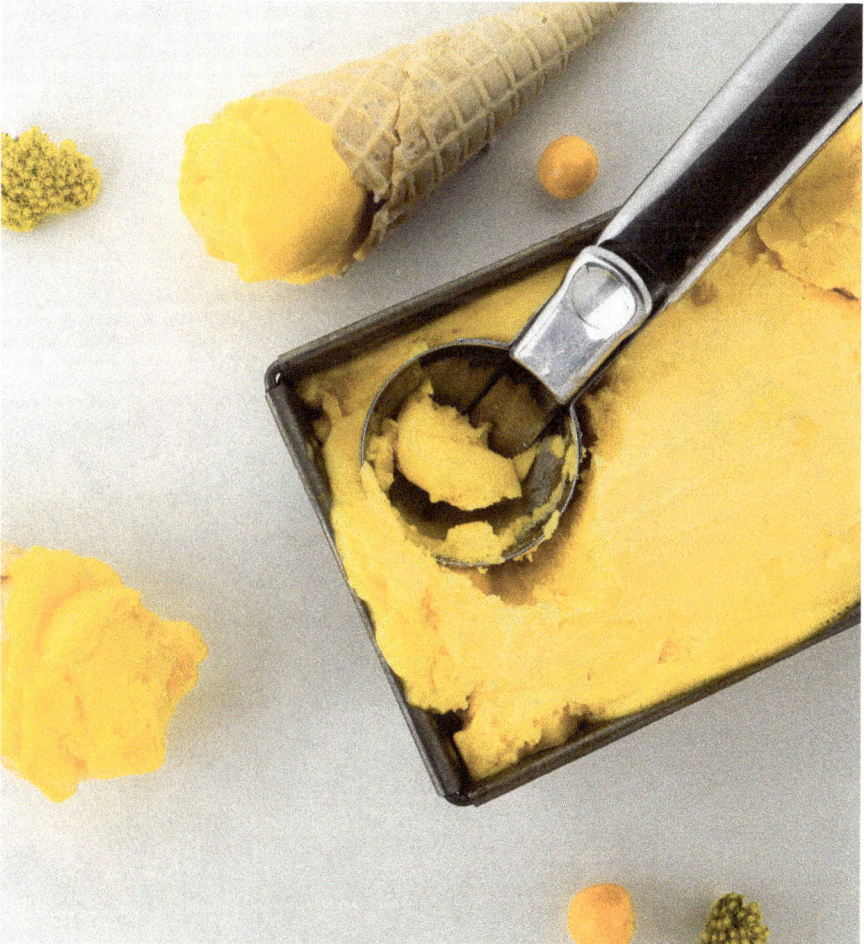

49. APPLE YOGURT WITH RAISINS

Cal.: 120 | Fat: 12g | Protein: 3g

Preparation Time: 11 minutes
Cooking Time: 4 hours
Servings: 4

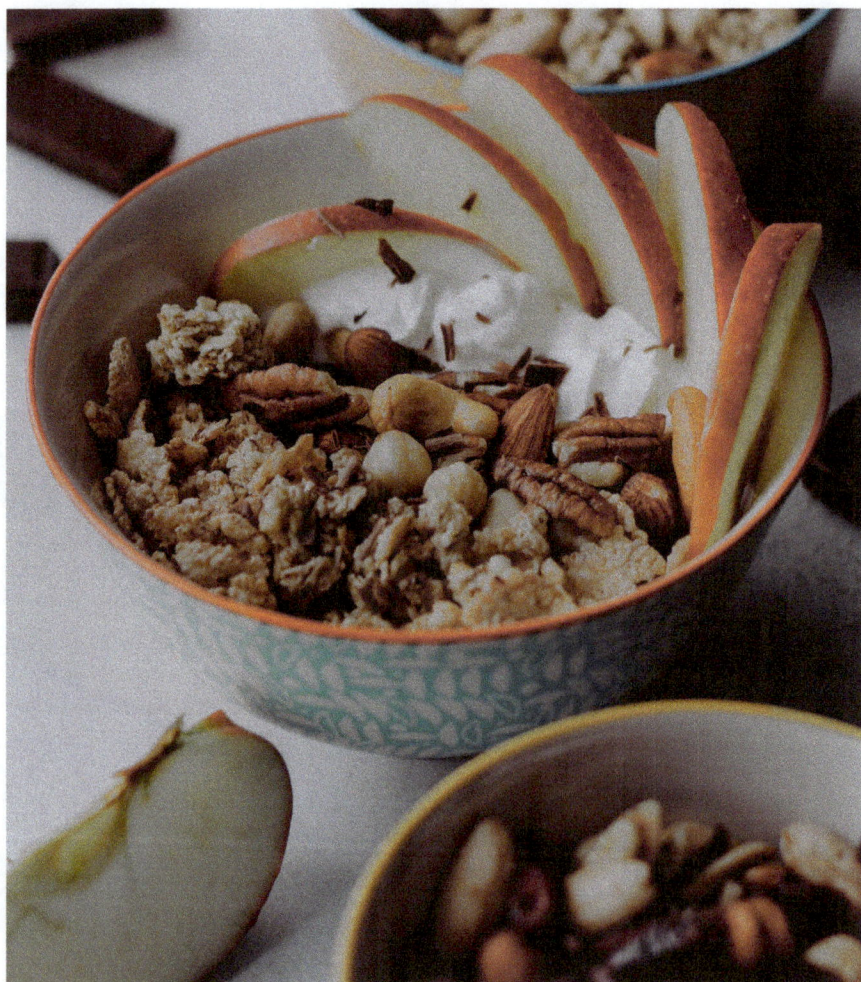

Ingredients

4 cups milk
½ cup Greek yogurt
½ cup sweet apples, peeled, cored and chopped
into small pieces
1 tsp. cinnamon
4 tsp. small raisins
2 tbsp. honey

Directions

1. Pour the milk into a pan and heat it to 180°F/82°C.

2. Cool it down to the room temperature.

3. Preheat the water bath to 113°F/45°C.

4. Mix in the yogurt, add the apples, cinnamon, honey, raisins and pour the mixture into canning jars.

5. Cover the jars with the lids and cook in the water bath for 3 hours.

6. When the time is up, cool down the jars to the room temperature and then refrigerate before serving.

50. DOCE DE BANANA

Cal.: 273 | Fat: 18g | Protein: 32g

Preparation Time: 10 minutes
Cooking Time: 45 minutes
Servings: 4

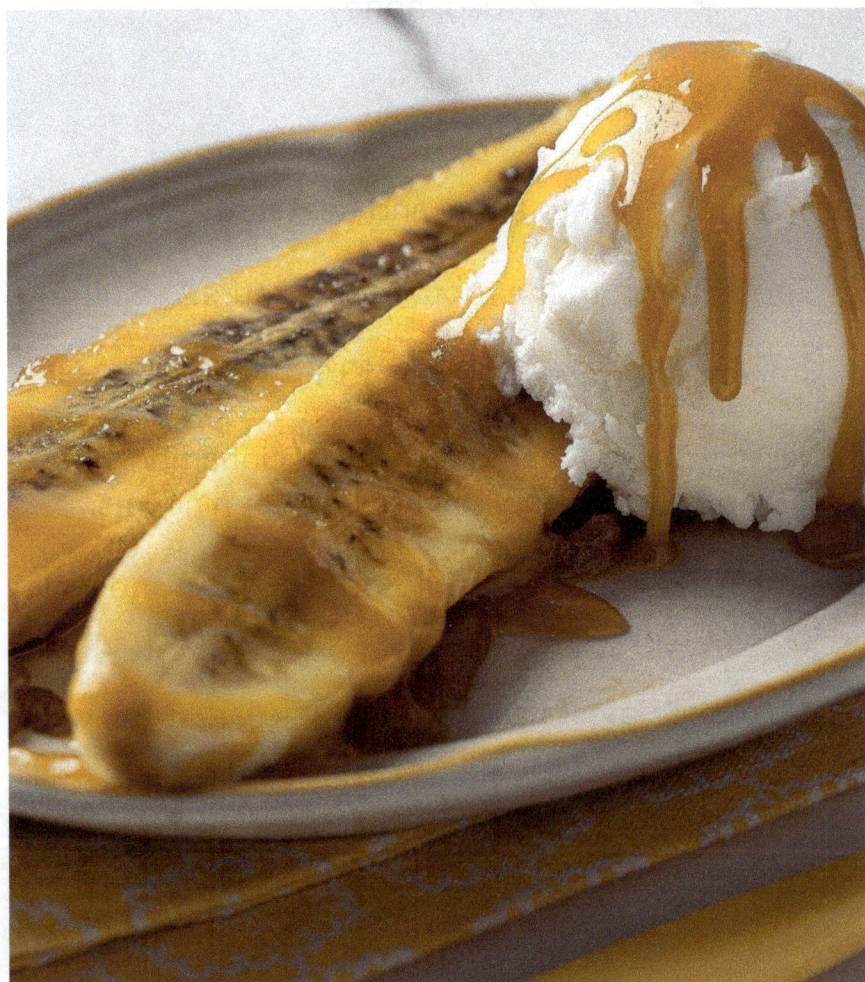

Ingredients

1 cup brown sugar
5 small bananas, peeled and cut to chunks
6 whole cloves
2 cinnamon sticks
Whipped cream

Directions

1. Preheat the Sous Vide machine to 176°F/80°C.

2. Combine the cloves, cinnamon sticks, brown sugar and banana. Place the mixture into a Ziploc bag and seal using the water immersion method.

3. Place the bag into the water bath. Cook in the cooker for 40 minutes.

4. Once done, remove the bag from the water bath and set aside to cool slightly.

5. Remove the cloves and cinnamon sticks and pour the remaining contents in a bowl. Top with whipped cream before serving.

TEMPERATURE CHARTS

🥩 MEAT	°F🌡 TEMPERA-TURE	⏱ TIME
Beef Steak, rare	129 °F	1 hour 30 min.
Beef Steak, medium-rare	136 °F	1 hour 30min.
Beef Steak, well done	158 °F	1 hour 30min.
Beef Roast, rare	133 °F	7 hours
Beef Roast, medium-rare	140 °F	6 hours
Beef Roast, well done	158 °F	5 hours
Beef Tough Cuts, rare	136 °F	24 hours
Beef Tough Cuts, medium-rare	149 °F	16 hours
Beef Tough Cuts, well done	185 °F	8 hours
Lamb Tenderloin, Rib eye, T-bone, Cutlets	134 °F	4 hours
Lamb Roast, Leg	134 °F	10 hours
Lamb Flank Steak, Brisket	134 °F	12 hours
Pork Chop, rare	136 °F	1 hour
Pork Chop, medium-rare	144 °F	1 hour
Pork Chop, well done	158 °F	1 hour
Pork Roast, rare	136 °F	3 hours

🥩 MEAT	°F🌡 TEMPERA-TURE	⏱ TIME
Pork Roast, medium-rare	144 °F	3 hours
Pork Roast, well done	158 °F	3 hours
Pork Tough Cuts, rare	144 °F	16 hours
Pork Tough Cuts, medium-rare	154 °F	12 hours
Pork Tough Cuts, well done	154 °F	8 hours
Pork Tenderloin	134 °F	1 hour 30min
Pork Baby Back Ribs	165 °F	6 hours
Pork Cutlets	134 °F	5 hours
Pork Spare Ribs	160 °F	12 hours
Pork Belly (quick)	185 °F	5 hours
Pork Belly (slow)	167 °F	24 hours

🐟 FISH AND SEAFOOD	°F🌡 TEMPERA-TURE	⏱ TIME
Fish, tender	104 °F	40 min.
Fish, tender and flaky	122 °F	40 min.
Fish, well done	140 °F	40 min.
Salmon, Tuna, Trout, Mackerel, Halibut, Snapper, Sole	126 °F	30 min.
Lobster	140 °F	50 min.
Scallops	140 °F	50 min.
Shrimp	140 °F	35 min.

🍗 POULTRY	🌡 TEMPERA-TURE	⏱ TIME
Chicken White Meat, super-supple	140 °F	2 hours
Chicken White Meat, tender and juicy	149 °F	1 hour
Chicken White Meat, well done	167 °F	1 hour
Chicken Breast, bone-in	146 °F	2 hours 30 min.
Chicken Breast, boneless	146 °F	1 hour
Turkey Breast, bone-in	146 °F	4 hours
Turkey Breast, boneless	146 °F	2 hours 30 min.
Duck Breast	134 °F	1 hour 30 min.
Chicken Dark Meat, tender	149 °F	1 hour 30 min.
Chicken Dark Meat, falling off the bone	167 °F	1 hour 30 min.
Chicken Leg or Thigh, bone-in	165 °F	4 hours
Chicken Thigh, boneless	165 °F	1 hour
Turkey Leg or Thigh	165 °F	2 hours
Duck Leg	165 °F	8 hours
Split Game Hen	150 °F	6 hours

🥕 VEGETABLES	°F🌡 TEMPERA-TURE	🕐 TIME
Vegetables, root (carrots, potato, parsnips, beets, celery root, turnips)	183 °F	3 hours
Vegetables, tender (asparagus, broccoli, cauliflower, fennel, onions, pumpkin, eggplant, green beans, corn)	183 °F	1 hour
Vegetables, greens (kale, spinach, collard greens, Swiss chard)	183 °F	3 min.

🍎 FRUITS	°F🌡 TEMPERA-TURE	🕐 TIME
Fruit, firm (apple, pear)	183 °F	45 min.
Fruit, for purée	185 °F	30 min.
Fruit, berries for topping desserts (blueberries, blackberries, raspberries, strawberries, cranberries)	154 °F	30 min.

WHAT TEMPERATURE SHOULD BE USED?

The rule of thumb is that the thicker the piece, the longer it should cook. Higher temperatures shorten the cooking time. Lower temperatures may take longer.

	TEMPERA-TURE	MIN COOK-ING TIME	MAX COOK-ING TIME
EGGS			
Soft Yolk	140°F (60°C)	1 hour	1 hour
Creamy Yolk	145°F (63°C)	¾ hour	1 hour
GREEN VEGETABLES			
Rare	183°F (84°C)	¼ hour	¾ hour
ROOTS			
Rare	183°F (84°C)	1 hour	3 hours
FRUITS			
Warm	154°F (68°C)	1¾ hour	2½ hour
Soft Fruits	185°F (85°C)	½ hour	1½ hour

	TEMPERA-TURE	MIN COOK-ING TIME	MAX COOK-ING TIME
CHICKEN			
Rare	140°F (60°C)	1 hour	3 hours
Medium	150°F (65°C)	1 hour	3 hours
Well Done	167°F (75°C)	1 hour	3 hours
BEEF STEAK			
Rare	130°F (54°C)	1½ hours	3 hours
Medium	140°F (60°C)	1½ hours	3 hours
Well Done	145°F (63°C)	1½ hours	3 hours
ROAST BEEF			
Rare	133°F (54°C)	7 hours	16 hours
Medium	140°F (60°C)	6 hours	14 hours
Well Done	158°F (70°C)	5 hours	11 hours
PORK CHOP BONE-IN			
Rare	136°F (58°C)	1 hour	4 hours
Medium	144°F (62°C)	1 hour	4 hours
Well Done	158°F (70°C)	1 hour	4 hours
PORK LOIN			
Rare	136°F (58°C)	3 hours	5½ hours
Medium	144°F (62°C)	3 hours	5 hours
Well Done	158°F (70°C)	3 hours	3½ hours
FISH			
Tender	104°F (40°C)	½ hour	½ hour
Medium	124°F (51°C)	½ hour	1 hour
Well Done	131°F (55°C)	½ hour	1½ hours

COOKING CONVERSION

TEMPERATURE CONVERSIONS	
CELSIUS	**FAHRENHEIT**
54.5°C	130°F
60.0°C	140°F
65.5°C	150°F
71.1°C	160°F
76.6°C	170°F
82.2°C	180°F
87.8°C	190°F
93.3°C	200°F
100°C	212°F

WEIGHT COVERSION	
½ oz.	15g
1 oz.	30g
2 oz.	60g
3 oz.	85g
4 oz.	110g
5 oz.	140g
6 oz.	170g
7 oz.	200g
8 oz.	225g
9 oz.	255g
10 oz.	280g
11 oz.	310g
12 oz.	340g
13 oz.	370g
14 oz.	400g
15 oz.	425g
1 lb.	450g

LIQUID VOLUME CONVERSION		
CUPS / TABLE-SPOONS	**FL. OUNCES**	**MILLILITERS**
1 cup	8 fl. Oz.	240 ml
¾ cup	6 fl. Oz.	180 ml
2/3 cup	5 fl. Oz.	150 ml
½ cup	4 fl. Oz.	120 ml
1/3 cup	2 ½ fl. Oz.	75 ml
¼ cup	2 fl. Oz.	60 ml
1/8 cup	1 fl. Oz.	30 ml
1 tablespoon	½ fl. Oz.	15 ml

TEASPOON (tsp.) / TABLESPOON (Tbsp.)	**MILLILITERS**
1 tsp.	5ml
2 tsp.	10ml
1 Tbsp.	15ml
2 Tbsp.	30ml
3 Tbsp.	45ml
4 Tbsp.	60ml
5 Tbsp.	75ml
6 Tbsp.	90ml
7 Tbsp.	105ml

LIQUID VOLUME MEASUREMENTS			
TABLE-SPOONS	TEASPOONS	FLUID OUNCES	CUPS
16	48	8 fl. Oz.	1
12	36	6 fl. Oz.	¾
8	24	4 fl. Oz.	½
5 ½	16	2 2/3 fl. Oz.	1/3
4	12	2 fl. Oz.	¼
1	3	0.5 fl. Oz.	1/16

RECIPE INDEX